THE ETHICS OF ARTIFICAL UTERUSES

Ectogenesis, the gestation of the foetus outside of the human body, will not for much longer be in the realm of science fiction; a number of projects attempting to develop ectogenetic technology are currently under way. This book examines the ethical implications of the development of ectogenesis.

Examining the implications for abortion ethics in particular, this book also deals with the ethical objections to developing such a technology and the uses to which it may be put, such as creating embryos to supply donor organs for transplantation. The development of the artificial uterus may well be similar to cloning: a sudden technological advance with dramatic ethical implications, thrust suddenly into the public eye.

ASHGATE STUDIES IN APPLIED ETHICS

Scandals in medical research and practice; physicians unsure how to manage new powers to postpone death and reshape life; business people operating in a world with few borders; damage to the environment; concern with animal welfare – all have prompted an international demand for ethical standards which go beyond matters of personal taste and opinion.

The *Ashgate Studies in Applied Ethics* series presents leading international research on the most topical areas of applied and professional ethics. Focusing on professional, business, environmental, medical and bio-ethics, the series draws from many diverse interdisciplinary perspectives including: philosophical, historical, legal, medical, environmental and sociological. Exploring the intersection of theory and practice, books in this series will prove of particular value to researchers, students, and practitioners worldwide.

Series Editors:

Ruth Chadwick, Director of ESRC Centre for Economic
and Social Aspects of Genomics (CESAGen) and Professor of Bioethics,
Lancaster University, UK
Dr David Lamb, Honorary Reader in Bioethics, University of Birmingham, UK
Professor Michael Davis, Center for the Study of Ethics in the Professions,
Illinois Institute of Technology, USA

The Ethics of Artificial Uteruses
Implications for Reproduction and Abortion

STEPHEN COLEMAN
Centre for Applied Philosophy
and Public Ethics
Charles Sturt University

ASHGATE

Published by
Ashgate Publishing Limited
Gower House
Croft Road
Aldershot
Hants GU11 3HR
England

Ashgate Publishing Company
Suite 420
101 Cherry Street
Burlington
Vermont, 05401–4405
USA

Ashgate website: http://www.ashgate.com

British Library Cataloguing in Publication Data
Coleman, Stephen
    The Ethics of Artificial Uteruses: Implications for Reproduction and Abortion.
    – (Ashgate Studies in Applied Ethics)
    1. Human reproductive technology – Moral and ethical aspects. 2. Human reproduction – Moral and ethical aspects. 3. Abortion – Moral and ethical aspects. Fetus – Legal status, laws, etc. I. Title.
    176

US Library of Congress Cataloging in Publication Data
Coleman, Stephen, 1937–
    The ethics of Artificial Uteruses: Implications for Reproduction and Abortion / Stephen Coleman.
        p.   cm.
    Includes bibliographical references and index.
    1. Ectogenesis – Moral and ethical aspects. 2. Human reproductive technology – Moral and ethical aspects. 3. Abortion – Moral and ethical aspects. I. Title.
    RG133.5.C654 2005
    176–dc22   2004007476

ISBN 0 7546 5051 0
This book is printed on acid free paper.
Printed and bound in Great Britain by Antony Rowe Ltd, Chippenham, Wiltshire

Contents

Preface and Acknowledgments

My interest in artificial uteruses first arose during my time as an undergraduate at Macquarie University in Sydney. I was studying a subject in Applied Ethics, during which I examined the problem of abortion. It was pointed out during a lecture that arguments in favour of abortion only allowed a woman to demand the removal of the foetus from her uterus, and not its death. If ectogenesis was to be developed, then this would significantly change the abortion debate. The topic was too large to be considered for my Honours thesis, but eventually became the topic of my PhD thesis. The examiners of that PhD enthusiastically recommended publication as a monograph. The end result is this book.

The material in Chapter 4 on general objections to reproductive technology began life as a paper I wrote entitled 'Surrogacy and the Artificial Uterus'. It was presented in this form at the International Conference on Applied Ethics at the Chinese University of Hong Kong in December 1999, before being modified and published as 'A Surrogate for Surrogacy? – The Artificial Uterus' in the *Australian Journal of Professional and Applied Ethics*, Vol. 1 (1999), pp. 49–60. This chapter benefited from the insightful comments of the participants of that conference, and the anonymous referees of the journal. The basic ideas from Chapter 7 have also seen life as a conference paper, being presented at The End of Natural Motherhood conference (hosted by The Ethics Centre at Oklahoma State University) in Tulsa, Oklahoma, in February 2002. Various comments made by participants at that conference were incorporated into the paper before it was published as 'Abortion and the Artificial Uterus' in the *Australian Journal of Professional and Applied Ethics*, Vol. 4 (2002,) pp. 9–18.

Both the PhD research upon which this book is based, and the preparation of the final manuscript, were supported by the Centre for Applied Philosophy and Public Ethics at Charles Sturt University. The book would not have been completed without that valuable support, and so I would like to thank the Director of the Centre, Seumas Miller, for his encouragement. I must also thank Barbara Nunn, a research assistant at the Centre, for proofreading the manuscript and preparing the camera ready copy.

There are many other people who I must thank for all the time, effort, and helpful advice that they gave me during the course of my research. My PhD supervisors at Monash University in Melbourne, Chin Liew Ten and Jeanette Kennett gave generously of their time and wisdom, and the original thesis would never have been completed without their invaluable assistance and encouragement. The markers of that thesis, Mary Anne Warren (San Francisco State University) and Arthur Kuflik (University of Vermont) also made many useful suggestions that have been incorporated into the text. Another person who has earned my undying gratitude is Catriona Mackenzie of Macquarie University in Sydney, who taught the Applied Ethics subject that first interested me in this topic, supervised my

Honours thesis, advised me on my choice of post-graduate department, and gave valuable comments on Chapter 6. Special thanks also to Michael Davis, Director of the Center for the Study of Ethics in the Professions at Illinois Institute of Technology, who read over the final manuscript of this book and gave me a great deal of valuable advice.

Thank you also to my children, Hannah and Jacqueline, who never stopped encouraging me by asking when my book would be finished, and whose surprising insights provoked me to deeper levels of thought on several issues.

Finally, and most importantly, thank you from the bottom of my heart, to my wife Nikki, who debated, discussed, proofread, babysat, encouraged and gave of her time, energy and health in every way possible to ensure that I would finally finish this work. I had the ideas for the book, but you had the energy and the commitment that ensured it actually happened. This book is for you.

Chapter 1

Ectogenesis: Why the Fuss?

In their book, *The Reproduction Revolution* Peter Singer and Deane Wells tell the story of Kim Bland, a baby born in 1981 weighing only 470 grams and nearly three months premature.[1] Though he had his problems in his early life, he survived. Singer and Wells note that 'He was the smallest baby to have survived at the Queen Victoria Medical Centre, and one of the smallest anywhere in the world.'[2] As we enter the new millennium, such cases are no longer rare. These cases show that the human foetus[3] no longer needs to spend anywhere near the traditional nine months inside the mother's uterus. With foetal viability being pushed back at such a rate, it seems likely that at some time in the not too distant future, a child will be born that has not spent any time at all in its mother's uterus – the first ectogenetic child.

Ectogenesis;[4] literally 'external origin' or 'outside creation'. The term is commonly used to refer to any device or process that would allow a foetus to develop to maturity without having to spend any time inside the body of a woman. This could be some sort of artificial uterine machine (probably similar in some ways to existing technologies such as humidicribs), a normal uterus removed from a woman's body and artificially nourished in an external environment, or even the use of the uterus *in situ* of one of the larger domestic animals, such as a cow or donkey. For the purposes of this discussion, I will consider only the first two types of ectogenesis, which are essentially indistinguishable in ethical terms.[5] The ethical

---

[1] Singer, Peter and Wells, Deane, *The Reproduction Revolution: New Ways of Making Babies*, (Oxford: Oxford University, 1984). Revised North American edition published as *Making Babies: The New Science and Ethics of Conception*, (New York: Scribners, 1985). The story of Kim Bland can be found on p. 131 of the Oxford edition.

[2] *Ibid.*

[3] This term is unfortunately spelt differently in different places. I have decided that in this book, I will spell it 'foetus'.

[4] Ectogenesis has also been called *in vitro* gestation (IVG) by Julien S. Murphy in 'Is Pregnancy Necessary? Feminist Concerns about Ectogenesis', *Hypatia*, 3 (1989), pp. 65–84 and external means of gestation by Frances Kamm in *Creation and Abortion*, (Oxford: Oxford University, 1992). For the purposes of this discussion, I will generally use the term ectogenesis, (or ectogenetic device) even when referring to the work of Murphy and Kamm, though where specific types of ectogenesis are referred to, I will on occasion use more specific terms. The meaning of these terms will be explained at that time.

[5] In suggesting that these two types of ectogenetic device are ethically indistinguishable, I am assuming that consent for the use of uterine materials has been obtained from the women donating these tissues, which has not always been the case in the past.

issues arising from the use of animals to gestate human foetuses are beyond the scope of this book. I would note however, that virtually all ethical issues that apply to the use of other ectogenetic methods would apply to the use of xeno-ectogenesis; there are simply additional issues that arise from the use of animals.

Why is ectogenesis important? Isn't it simply another form of IVF? The answer to this is, certainly, no. While other extensions of IVF technology, such as GIFT (gamete intra-fallopian transfer), or ET (embryo transfer), raise few new ethical issues, the implications of ectogenesis are far more important. The most important theoretical application of ectogenesis is in the area of abortion. It has been suggested for some time now, that the right to abortion only entitles the woman to evacuation of the uterus, and not to secure the death of the foetus. This suggestion I shall call severance theory, following Leslie Cannold.[6] Prominent among severance theorists are writers such as Judith Jarvis Thomson[7] and Christine Overall.[8] If severance theory is correct, then the development of ectogenesis might dramatically change the landscape of the abortion arguments, by allowing the separation of two currently inseparable events, the evacuation of the foetus from the uterus, and the death of the foetus. While the most important ethical implications of ectogenesis arise out of the arguments surrounding abortion, this is certainly not the only ethical issue arising from the development of ectogenesis. The development of such technology would also have implications in the treatment of infertility, and in the area of transplant surgery.

In evaluating the ethical implications of human ectogenesis, I shall first examine the current state of play on ectogenetic research, both from a scientific and legal perspective. This discussion is the basis of Chapter 2. In Chapter 3 I will then outline the theoretical basis with which I will be working, and will briefly discuss some arguments that have been proposed in favour of pursuing research into ectogenesis. Chapter 4 examines some objections that have been proposed against the development and use of ectogenesis, and attempts to evaluate the strength of those objections.

Chapter 5 introduces the issue of abortion, and contains a detailed analysis of severance theory arguments on abortion, and the implications of ectogenesis for these arguments. My conclusion in this chapter is that the morality of abortion cannot be decided without reference to the moral status of the embryo and foetus. Chapter 6 is thus an examination of this topic, in which I examine the major positions on moral status, and draw conclusions regarding the status of the embryo and foetus. Chapter 7 returns to the issue of abortion, re-examining the implications of ectogenesis on the abortion debate in light of the conclusion on moral status found in Chapter 6. Chapter 8 moves on from the abortion debate to examine the issues arising from the use of ectogenesis to create embryos as organ

---

[6] *The Abortion Myth: Feminism, Morality and the Hard Choices Women Make*, (St Leonards: Allen & Unwin, 1998).
[7] 'A Defence of Abortion', *Philosophy and Public Affairs*, 1 (1971), pp. 47–66.
[8] See *Ethics and Human Reproduction: A Feminist Analysis*, (Boston: Allen & Unwin, 1987).

donors for transplant surgery. Chapter 9 draws the final conclusions, and contains recommendations for the regulation of the use of ectogenetic technology.

Chapter 2

The Current State of Play

Scientific Aspects

Is ectogenesis merely science fiction, or could it soon become scientific fact? This is a difficult question to answer, since scientific research often travels along unusual paths. In this particular case, it would seem that there are two ways in which ectogenesis might be achieved: the direct research method, and the indirect research method. Direct research into an artificial uterus, and more importantly an artificial placenta, started in the 1950s, and continues in a few research establishments today. If ectogenesis is to be achieved, however, it seems more likely that the most important breakthroughs will come through indirect research. There are two main branches of research that seem most relevant in this case: research aimed at solving the problems of human infertility, and research aimed at improving the survival rates of premature births. These two types of research are both major fields of medical study, so I will examine them separately, to see what the implications for ectogenetic research are.

Research on Infertility

The possibilities of achieving the fertilisation of an egg outside the body has fascinated the medical community for many years. Attempts were made to fertilise animal eggs in the laboratory as long ago as 1878, though success was not achieved until 1934.[1] In 1944 John Rock of Harvard University successfully fertilised a human egg with sperm *in vitro*. To prove that such attempts had achieved genuine fertilisation, in 1959 a fertilised rabbit egg was inserted into the uterus of a second rabbit, resulting in pregnancy.[2] The first human pregnancy through *In Vitro* Fertilisation (IVF) was achieved in 1973, in Melbourne, but unfortunately this pregnancy lasted only nine days.[3] Success was not far away though, and one of the definitive moments in modern medicine occurred in England on 25 July 1978, when Louise Brown, the first 'test-tube baby', was born.

---

[1] See Paul J. Jersild, 'On Having Children: A Theological and Moral Analysis of *In Vitro* Fertilisation', in Edward D. Schneider (ed.), *Questions About the Beginning of Life*, (Minneapolis: Augsburg, 1985), p. 31.
[2] *Ibid.*
[3] David deKretser et. al., 'Transfer of a Human Zygote', *The Lancet*, 2 (1973), pp. 728–9.

Before Louise Brown, human life had only ever begun in the uterus; after Louise Brown, a major step towards ectogenesis had been taken.

Human life could now begin in the laboratory, but for how long could that life be maintained outside the human body? Conception and initial growth can occur in a petri-dish, but if the fertilised egg is to survive, it must be transferred out of the petri-dish and into a uterus, within two or three days. After about three days *in vitro,* the embryo has divided to 32 cells. While no pregnancy has been recorded from an embryo larger than this, it is possible to keep the embryo growing longer in the petri-dish. In 1975, Robert Edwards managed to keep one embryo alive for nine days, before he decided to prepare it for dissection, worried that it would die before he managed to examine it:

> The embryo was still a speck, only just visible in our culture dish, but for me it represented the crucial stages of human embryology, the actual moments when the foundations are being laid for the formation of the body's organs. Cells and tissues grew and moved, assuming new forms in readiness for the moment when the embryo would begin to take a recognisable shape. Normally, of course, the embryo would be developing in this way inside its mother's womb, but I was privileged to watch it in our culture dish with all its promise of future growth.[4]

Edwards never managed to repeat his success, but another physiologist, Dennis New, has managed to keep mouse and rat embryos alive for approximately two weeks.[5] Given the differences in gestational periods, this would equate to about four weeks of human pregnancy, since after two weeks the rodent embryos have developed all their organs and the placenta.

So it is clear that human life no longer needs to begin inside the human body. For half of the first week of life, the embryo can live just as well in a dish in the laboratory, as inside its mother's body. But what about the other end of the pregnancy?

Research on Foetal Viability[6]   When the US Supreme Court brought down its ruling in the famous case of *Roe* v *Wade* in 1973, it drew a legal line at the point of foetal viability.[7] They defined viability as the point at which the foetus is

---

[4] Robert Edwards, *A Matter of Life*, (London: Sphere, 1981), p. 131.
[5] Peter Singer and Deane Wells, *The Reproduction Revolution: New Ways of Making Babies,* (Oxford: Oxford University, 1984), p. 133.
[6] This section, and the following section on the care of premature newborns, draws heavily on V.Y.H. Yu, 'Prematurity and Low Birth Weight', in Robinson and Roberton (eds), *Practical Paediatrics*, 4th ed., (Edinburgh: Churchill Livingstone, 1998); V.Y.H. Yu 'Improving the Outcome of Preterm and Low Birthweight Infants', Unpublished manuscript, (1995); and my own personal discussions with Victor Yu, Professor of Neonatology and Director of Neonatal Intensive Care, Monash Medical Centre. While his help was invaluable, obviously any mistakes or omissions are solely my responsibility.
[7] In this case, possibly the most famous legal ruling in history, the US Supreme Court ruled that prior to the end of the first trimester any decisions regarding abortion must be left up to

potentially able to live outside its mother's uterus, albeit with artificial aid. It noted that viability is usually placed at about seven months, or 28 weeks, although it may occur earlier, even at 24 weeks. Twenty-five years later, things have changed quite significantly. When *Roe* v *Wade* was handed down, 28 weeks was commonly used as the cut off point for treatment. Foetuses born earlier than this were often given only palliative care, but were not given active treatment, as it was known that at that time there was nothing that could be done to save them. These days, things have changed so much that in the Neonatal Intensive Care Unit (NICU) of the Monash Medical Centre in Melbourne, 28 weeks is considered to be the 90-95 per cent survival point. At this NICU, the survival of babies born at only 24 weeks gestation was routine, and the survival of babies born at only 23 weeks was not unknown. Even more surprisingly, few of these babies have significant disabilities.

Thus in 25 years, the age of viability has been lowered by four weeks. Though *Roe* v *Wade* noted that the age of viability can sometimes be as early as 24 weeks, this was considered absolutely extreme at the time. The death of babies born at 28 weeks was expected, and the vast majority of survivors would be severely disabled. Perhaps the most interesting part about this reduction, at least as far as ectogenesis is concerned, is that most of the reduction in the age of viability is attributable to new techniques that attempt, as far as possible, to mimic the uterine environment. Given that medical science has found that in most cases the best results are obtained from such techniques, can more direct research into an artificial placenta and uterus be far away?

The main functions of the placenta prior to birth are oxygenation of and supply of nutrients to the foetal blood, and the removal of waste products from that blood. The amniotic fluid acts to regulate foetal temperature, to prevent dehydration, and as a barrier to infection. When treating extremely premature newborns, neonatologists attempt to mimic the uterine function when treating problems of these types. They have been largely successful in doing so, except in the case of oxygenation of the foetal blood. This was the subject of many direct experiments in the 1960s and 1970s, and will be dealt with in the later section on direct experimentation.

Care of Extremely Premature Newborns Extremely premature infants are commonly unable to derive adequate nutrition through normal oral feeding. This is due to a combination of several factors, including a poor suck reflex, uncoordinated swallowing and the immaturity of the intestinal tract. Thus neonatologists must often resort to parenteral feeding – delivering nutrition directly into the bloodstream by means of an IV drip. The nutrition thus delivered is also

the pregnant woman and her attending physician. From the end of the first trimester to the end of the second trimester, the State may regulate abortions in ways that are reasonably related to maternal health. After the end of the second trimester, at the point of viability, the State may regulate or even proscribe abortion except where it is medically necessary to protect the life or health of the mother. A detailed legal and philosophical discussion of the case can be found in Ronald Dworkin, *Life's Dominion*, (London: HarperCollins, 1995).

specially tailored to produce minimum waste products, thus reducing the likelihood of problems in the newborns equally immature renal system. Sensors are placed on the skin of the premature infant to directly measure chemical levels in the blood, so that any imbalances can be quickly corrected. Thus in both the maintenance of adequate nutrition, and the control of waste products, the neonatologist is attempting to mimic the actions of the placenta, rather than trying to utilise the normal body systems, as would be the case when treating an adult or small child.

The immaturity of the skin of the premature infant is also a problem that the neonatologist must deal with. While many people now realise that the skin is an organ, the importance of that organ is usually not so recognised. However, when dealing with a premature infant, when that organ is immature, the importance of the skin becomes apparent. The immaturity of the premature infant's skin (which has been equated to a third degree burn in an adult) leads to serious problems in dehydration, and resistance to infection, as well as contributing to problems in temperature control. The reduced amount of subcutaneous fat in premature infants is another contributing factor in these problems, especially the problem of temperature control. In a uterine environment, these problems would be dealt with by the amniotic fluid, so medical science has discovered that the best way to combat these problems in premature infants is to try to mimic the uterine environment as much as possible. Thus premature infants are usually placed in a humidicrib. As its name suggests, this special crib maintains a humid environment around the infant (usually about 90 per cent humidity) as well as maintaining a constant warm temperature. This prevents both dehydration and hypothermia. Some attempts have even been made to place the premature infant in an artificial amniotic fluid, but this has proven impractical, for a number of reasons. These include difficulties in accessing the infant for treatment, and problems in maintaining respiration while in the fluid. However, some neonatologists have placed fatty liquids or creams on the skin of premature infants, thus creating a thin 'amniotic layer' as a barrier against infection. Again it can be seen that the neonatologist has generally tried to mimic the uterine environment, rather than relying solely on the normal body systems, as would be the case with an adult.

Virtually all premature infants have respiratory problems. Treatment for such problems ideally begins before birth, with the mother being given an injection of corticosteroids, which are known to cross the placenta, and greatly accelerate lung development.[8] After birth, respiratory problems are treated with artificial ventilation. The ventilators that are commonly used on adults have been shown to damage infant lungs, so special high frequency oscillation ventilators are commonly used. These ventilators supply an equivalent volume of air to conventional ventilators, but do so by providing an enormous number of relatively small breaths, rather than a smaller number of large breaths (high frequency oscillation ventilators use breath rates of between 600 and 900 breaths per minute,

---

[8] If an injection of corticosteroids is given enough time to work (generally at least 24 hours) then it can advance organ development by as much as a week.

as opposed to about 100 breaths per minute with conventional ventilation). Used in combination with the ventilator, is surfactant replacement therapy, which has been described as 'the most exciting advance in neonatal medicine of the last decade'.[9] Surfactant is a naturally occurring chemical, which helps the lungs absorb oxygen. In premature infants, there is usually insufficient surfactant in the lungs, which leads to problems in the absorption of oxygen. Surfactant replacement therapy treats this problem by supplying synthetic surfactant directly to the lung surfaces. It is believed that up to half of the decline in the US national infant mortality death rate reported between 1989 and 1990 can be attributed to the introduction of surfactant therapy.[10]

The same skin surface monitors that are used to measure blood chemicals are used to check oxygen levels (actually the most important chemical level in the blood of the premature infant), to ensure that the infant is receiving the correct level of oxygen. Too little oxygen can quickly lead to permanent brain damage, but too much oxygen can also destroy some parts of the brain, as oxygen becomes toxic at higher concentrations.

The treatment of respiratory problems in premature infants is clearly quite different from the treatment of most other problems, as the treatment relies exclusively on the body system that is responsible for oxygenation of the blood after birth; the lungs. In most other neonatal problems, the treatment relies on mimicking the uterine environment, but this is not the case with treatment for respiratory problems. This is somewhat surprising, since artificial oxygenation of the blood was a major area of research in the 1960s and 1970s, as part of direct research attempts to develop an artificial placenta. To see why such research has proven largely unsuccessful, it will be necessary to look at that direct research.

Direct Research towards Ectogenesis (The Past)

In the 1950s and 1960s, there were a large number of groups performing experiments on artificial placentas and uteruses. Most of these groups used artificial perfusion techniques. Some seemed to be interested only in understanding the mechanics of the placenta,[11] but others were explicit in their intention to try to develop an artificial placenta.[12] Most of these studies saw the artificial placenta as

---

[9] V.Y.H. Yu, 'Improving the Outcome of Premature and Low Birthweight Infants', p. 3.

[10] *Ibid.*

[11] See for example Walter R. Groeber, 'Antiabruption Dynamics of the Intervillous Circulation in an Artificial Uterus', *American Journal of Obstetrics & Gynecology*, 95 (1966), pp. 640–47, or Kermit Krantz, Theodore Panos and James Evans, 'Physiology of Maternal–Foetal Relationship Through the Extracorporeal Circulation of the Human Placenta', *American Journal of Obstetrics & Gynecology*, 83 (1962), pp. 1214–28.

[12] John Callaghan and Jose Delos Angeles, 'Long Term Extracorporeal Circulation in the Development of an Artificial Placenta for Respiratory Distress of the Newborn', *Surgical Forum*, 12 (1961), pp. 215–17; John Callaghan et al., 'Study of Prepulmonary Bypass in the Development of an Artificial Placenta for Prematurity and Respiratory Distress Syndrome of

a means of supplementing the lungs in their attempts to provide oxygen to the body's tissues, though some appeared to be of the opinion that their artificial placenta would be capable of doing all the work of a real one, and thus suspended their subjects in an artificial amniotic fluid.[13] While most of these experiments succeeded in maintaining stable blood oxygen levels in their subjects for relatively short periods, attempts to keep the subject attached to the artificial placenta for longer periods inevitably resulted in death. The problems with the use of the artificial placenta (now commonly known as extracorporeal circulation) were detailed by Bartlett and Gazzaniga in 1978.[14] It was eventually discovered that extracorporeal membrane oxygenation (ECMO) could be used for partial respiratory support, without causing damage to the heart of the newborn.[15] ECMO was eventually brought into use to aid newborns with severe respiratory distress, having previously been used with success in adults with similar problems.[16] However, the technique no longer utilised the umbilical blood vessels, since better results were achieved using carotid arteries, and jugular and femoral veins.

the Newborn', *Journal of Thoracic and Cardiovascular Surgery*, 44 (1962), pp. 600–607; John Callaghan, Earl Maynes and Henry Hug, 'Studies on Lambs of the Development of an Artificial Placenta: Review of Nine Long–Term Survivors of Extracorporeal Circulation Maintained in a Fluid Medium', *Canadian Journal of Surgery*, 8 (1965), pp. 208–13; Geoffrey Chamberlain, 'An Artificial Placenta: The Development of an Extracorporeal System for Maintenance of Immature Infants with Respiratory Problems', *American Journal of Obstetrics & Gynecology*, 100 (1968), pp. 615–26; Amarendra SenGupta, Howard Taylor and Willem Kolff, 'An Artificial Placenta Designed to Maintain Life During Cardiorespiratory Distress', *Transactions: American Society for Artificial Internal Organs,*10 (1964), pp. 63–5; C.L. Sarin et al., 'Further Development of an Artificial Placenta with the use of Membrane Oxygenator and Venovenous Perfusion', *Surgery*, 60 (1966), pp. 754–60.
[13] Callaghan's first experiments (1961) used the artificial placenta as a supplement to normal respiration. In later experiments, his teams used the artificial placenta for all respiration of the subject, first by clamping the endotracheal tube (1962) and then by placing the subject in a fluid medium (1965). The suspension in artificial amniotic fluid was also the technique used by the team of Warren Zapol, who achieved the then record perfusion time of 55 hours. See Warren Zapol et al., 'Artificial Placenta: Two Days of Extrauterine Support of the Isolated Premature Lamb Foetus', *Science*, 166 (1969), pp. 617–18.
[14] R.H. Bartlett and A.B. Gazzaniga, 'Extracorporeal Circulation for Cardiopulmonary Failure', *Current Problems in Surgery*, 15 (1978), pp. 1–96.
[15] Bartley P. Griffith et al., 'Arteriovenous ECMO for Neonatal Respiratory Support: A Study in Perigestational Lambs', *The Journal of Thoracic and Cardiovascular Surgery*, 77 (1979), pp. 595–601.
[16] Warren Zapol et al., 'Extracorporeal Membrane Oxygenation in Severe Acute Respiratory Failure: A Randomised Prospective Study', *Journal of the American Medical Association*, 242 (1979), p. 2193.

Following extensive testing in clinical situations,[17] and a randomised trial,[18] ECMO eventually became an accepted technique in neonatal medicine. However, less than 15 years after its introduction, ECMO is now virtually obsolete in the treatment of premature infants. This is due to several factors, including the aforementioned introduction of surfactant therapy and high frequency oscillation ventilators. The biggest problem with the use of ECMO in the NICU, however, is its limited application. ECMO is contraindicated when the patient weighs less than 2 kilograms, since in smaller patients the blood vessels are too small to accept the large catheters required to maintain a sufficient blood flow through the ECMO circuit. Since virtually all extremely premature infants weigh less than 2 kilograms, these days the use of ECMO with infants is generally confined to the operating theatre, where it is used to maintain infant blood flow during major cardio-pulmonary surgery.

Direct Research towards Ectogenesis (Current)

Current direct research into ectogenesis can be divided into the same two types as indirect research – the first aimed at improving the survival rates of premature newborns, the second aimed at overcoming human infertility. However, I would differentiate the following research groups from those undertaking indirect research because the research undertaken by the groups I will be discussing attempts to use completely artificial means – either a completely artificial placenta, or a uterus (or uterine substitute) that is completely external to any human body.

Research Towards an Artificial Placenta to Combat Prematurity There have been few direct attempts to develop an artificial placenta since the 1960s; the most successful attempts have probably been made by the team led by Yoshinori Kuwabara in Tokyo. They are quite explicit in their aims: 'We have two objectives in our research. One is for animal models for foetal experimental medicine. The other is for clinical use, to rescue very immature or sick foetuses'.[19] Their best results, after many previous experiments,[20] used pancuronium bromide to suppress foetal movement and swallowing (which had been implicated in foetal death in the previous studies) and managed to incubate two goat foetuses, one for 494 hours (20.5 days), and the other for 542 hours (22.5 days). Both survived removal from

---

[17] Robert Bartlett et al., 'Extracorporeal Membrane Oxygenation for Newborn Respiratory Failure: Forty–five Cases', *Surgery*, 92 (1982), pp. 425–33.

[18] Robert Bartlett et al., 'Extracorporeal Circulation in Neonatal Respiratory Failure: A Prospective Randomised Study', *Pediatrics*, 76 (1985), pp. 479–87.

[19] Yoshinori Kuwabara, quoted in Peter Hadfield 'Japanese Pioneers Raise Kid in Rubber Womb' *New Scientist*, (25 April 1992), p. 5.

[20] Yoshinori Kuwabara et al., 'Development of Extrauterine Foetal Incubation System Using Extracorporeal Membrane Oxygenator', *Artificial Organs*, 11 (1987), pp. 224–7, p. 224 and Yoshinori Kuwabara et al., 'Artificial Placenta: Long–Term Extrauterine Incubation of Isolated Goat Foetuses', *Artificial Organs*, 13 (1989), pp. 527–31.

the apparatus,[21] and with ventilator support maintained stable blood gases for 704 hours and 169 hours (29 and 7 days) respectively. However, both died of respiratory insufficiency within hours of removal of ventilator support. The team note that there are still problems to be overcome, but 'foresee the clinical use of this kind of approach in premature neonates with severe organ immaturity or lung hypoplasia'.[22] Given that the smallest goat foetus that they have successfully incubated is a comparatively large 1.6 kilograms, there are obviously some problems that they do not mention, such as using ECMO on extremely small premature infants, in situations where it is currently contraindicated.

Research Towards an Artificial Uterus to Combat Prematurity The only research towards an artificial uterus designed to help premature infants that is currently underway, is the patented theoretical work of Dr William Cooper.[23] In 1991, Cooper filed a patent application for a 'placental chamber', which he suggests is capable of supporting the life of a prematurely-born baby. 'It is one object of this invention ... to provide a system which provides a foetus with an artificial environment which mimics the baby's pre-birth environment'.[24] The invention is a small chamber divided into two sections, the lower one filled with artificial amniotic fluid in which the 'patient' would float, and the upper part consisting of a shelf on which the foetus' natural placenta would rest. The foetus' umbilical cord would reach from the bottom section into the top section. Presumably, the placenta would then be artificially perfused, though there is no mention of this in the two descriptions of the device to which I have access. One does wonder how Cooper plans to deal with the major problem of removing the placenta intact from the mother's uterus, and with the mechanics of preventing foetal death while commencing perfusion of the placenta, all without allowing the foetus to take its first breath (which would make its later suspension in artificial amniotic fluid extremely difficult). It should be noted that Cooper is unique in the literature in believing that the foetus' natural placenta could form part of its life support system after removal from the mother's uterus.

Research Towards an Artificial Uterus to Combat Infertility The only research being undertaken in this area that I have been able to discover, is being undertaken by a team in Bologna, Italy, headed by Dr Carlo Bulletti. In 1988 this team published details of a study whereby surplus embryos from the university's IVF programme were implanted into artificially perfused uteri, obtained after removal

---

[21] The foetuses were both unable to stand or breathe by themselves, assumed to be an after-effect of the sedatives given during the experiment.
[22] *Ibid.*, p. 1002.
[23] Sabra Chartrand, 'Patents', *New York Times*, (19 July 1993) p. D2.
[24] Dr William Cooper, 'Placental Chamber – Artificial Uterus', United States Patent number 5,218,958, filed 21 February 1991; granted 15 June 1993; column 1. Quoted in Susan Merrill Squier, *Babies in Bottles: Twentieth–Century Visions of Reproductive Technology*, (New Brunswick: Rutgers, 1994), p. 97.

from women who required a hysterectomy due to cervical cancer.[25] It was noted in the article describing the experiment that 'the present study was undertaken to obtain the first early human pregnancy in vitro because future complete ectogenesis should not be ruled out'.[26] The experiment had the additional aim of improving understanding of the implantation of the human embryo into the endometrium, and thus giving a chance of increasing the success rate of implantation in the IVF programme. Bulletti and his team managed to get an embryo to implant in the wall of the artificially perfused uterus, and allowed it to grow there for 52 hours, before removing it for dissection. It should be noted that the limit of 52 hours was due to problems in the perfusion of the uterus, not any problems involving the embryos themselves.[27] While the team has not implanted any more embryos into the artificially perfused uteri, the possibility of continued research in this area certainly exists.

Summary

Research towards ectogenesis comes in two main forms. Direct research, in which ectogenesis of one form or another is the primary goal, and indirect research, where ectogenesis is a plausible side effect of research in others areas; specifically research into infertility, and research into the problems of prematurity.

Direct research was quite common in the 1950s and 1960s, but is relatively rare today. This may be because the previous research seemed to lead to something of a dead end, the technique of ECMO, which was to a large extent superseded soon after it was implemented. The few groups working on ectogenetic research today have achieved some successes in this area, though they obviously face problems in bringing any form of ectogenesis into reality. The work on artificially perfused human uteri seems stalemated, at least as far as ectogenesis goes, due to difficulties in maintaining a viable uterus outside the human body. Cooper's theoretical work seems to have major practical problems, especially the problem of removing the natural placenta intact from the maternal uterus. The work at the University of California seems mainly concerned with improving existing ECMO techniques. The work at the University of Tokyo has achieved results far beyond those achieved in the past, but there are problems with this research too, particularly in applying the results achieved with relatively mature goat foetuses to the much smaller premature human infant.

While the scientific work seems to be somewhat stalemated, none of the problems appear to be insurmountable. Indirect research has already reduced the amount of time that the foetus needs to spend in the maternal uterus, from the usual 40 weeks, down to about 23 weeks. Obviously the more effort that is put into research, and particularly into direct research, the more likely it is that the

[25] Carlo Bulletti et al., 'Early Human Pregnancy *in vitro* Utilising an Artificially Perfused Uterus', *Fertility and Sterility*, 49 (1988), pp. 991–6.
[26] *Ibid.*, p. 991.
[27] *Ibid.*, p. 995.

problems facing ectogenesis will be overcome. While at present it seems that ectogenesis in any form is still some way off, as we have seen with the rapid development of mammalian cloning, a breakthrough could come at any time.

Legal Aspects

Having made an examination of the current state of scientific research towards ectogenesis, I would now like to turn my attention to the current legal status of research in this area. In examining the scientific aspects of ectogenetic research, I noted that there two ways in which ectogenesis might be achieved; through direct research, and through indirect research. The legal aspects of ectogenetic research are similar, in that there are two types of research to which the law may apply. However, these are not direct and indirect research, but rather research into complete ectogenesis, and research into incomplete ectogenesis. Complete ectogenesis, in this context, involves taking a fertilised egg and implanting it into a device designed to carry the resulting foetus to term, while incomplete ectogenesis involves moving an existing foetus from its mother's uterus to another device that is designed to accept it, and carry it to term.

Generally speaking, it is complete ectogenesis that is the subject of legal sanction. The attempt to create a device that would allow reproduction without utilising the female reproductive tract is widely considered to be ethically suspect, and so laws against this practice are included in the statutes of many jurisdictions. Attempts to save premature foetuses, on the other hand, are not generally considered problematic, so incomplete ectogenesis is not subject to the same legal restrictions.

While the legal status of ectogenetic research is important, I do not want to spend too much time discussing the legal status of such research in every jurisdiction in the world. My approach will therefore be to examine only a sample of laws from various places around the world. I will first examine international laws and guidelines on this sort of research. Then I will examine the situation in the two countries which led the world for many years in the closely related field of IVF research; Australia and the United Kingdom (UK). These two countries provide a nice contrast, since one (the UK) is a single jurisdiction, and the other (Australia) is a multi-jurisdictional country, where both state and federal laws impact on the status of ectogenetic research. Finally I shall examine the situation in the United States, as this country is the largest medical researcher in the world. In examining the United States, I will not survey the laws in each of the 50 states, as this would be both unnecessary and time-consuming. Rather I shall simply examine the federal rulings on this matter. I should note that at this stage I am only examining the law as it relates to research on human embryos and foetuses. I will discuss animal research later.

Current Laws: International

There are no international laws, agreements or guidelines that cover research into ectogenesis. This is basically because there is a lack of international agreement on the ethics of any kind of foetal research. Guidelines on foetal and foetal tissue research are specifically excluded from the ethical guidelines of the Council for International Organizations of Medical Sciences (CIOMS) and the World Health Organization (WHO). In the Background Note issued with the *International Ethical Guidelines for Biomedical Research Involving Human Subjects*, Zbigniew Bankowski, the Secretary-General of CIOMS, writes:

> Certain areas of research do not receive special mention in these guidelines; they include human genetic research, embryo and foetal research, and foetal tissue research. These represent research areas in rapid evolution and in various respects controversial. The Steering Committee considered that since there is no universal agreement on all the ethical issues raised by these research areas it would be premature to try to cover them in the present guidelines.[28]

It does seem reasonable to suggest, however, that if there was disagreement about the ethics of ectogenesis, this disagreement would mainly concern complete ectogenesis. Attempts to save premature foetuses by means of incomplete ectogenesis do seem to fall within the principles expressed in the guidelines, since such research only involves attempts to save what are generally seen as existing lives.

Current Laws: Australia

In considering the legal position of ectogenetic research in Australia, there are two legal arenas that must be considered. First, there are the State Laws. Three of the six Australian states have passed specific Acts that contain provisions that would rule out ectogenetic research on humans; Victoria, South Australia and Western Australia, while the other three states rely on laws of precedent (which can include federal laws and recommendations). Second, there are the federal guidelines on the matter, which in this case means the semi-legal ethical guidelines issued by the National Health and Medical Research Council (NHMRC). The NHMRC is a federal statutory body, one of whose roles is to distribute federal research funds through grants to research programmes. Since federal funding is by far the largest source of funding for medical research in Australia, the NHMRC wields a great deal of power in determining the ethical standards of research in Australia. There are two NHMRC documents which relate to ectogenetic research, the NHMRC Statement on Human Experimentation and Supplementary notes, 1992 and the

---

[28] Zbigniew Bankowski, 'International Ethical Guidelines for Biomedical Research Involving Human Subjects', in *Ethics and Research on Human Subjects: International Guidelines,* Geneva: CIOMS, (1993), p. ix.

NHMRC Ethical Guidelines on Assisted Reproductive Technology, 1996. While these statements do not have any actual legal power, they are extremely important for two reasons. First, as the ethical pronouncements of a federal statutory body, they are treated with respect. Second, breach of the NHMRC guidelines for research may result in the withdrawal of federal funding for all research programmes at that research institution, so breach of the guidelines would only be countenanced by those who were working at an institution that had no current or future need for federal funding – an extremely rare situation.

Supplementary Note Four of the Statement on Human Experimentation concerns *in vitro* fertilisation and embryo transfer. Point Five notes that continuation of embryonic development beyond the stage at which implantation would normally occur is not acceptable. Section 11 of the Ethical Guidelines on Assisted Reproductive Technology lists prohibited/unacceptable practices. The second of these is culturing an embryo *in vitro* for more than 14 days. These statements would obviously rule out research into complete ectogenesis.

Current Laws: United Kingdom

In the United Kingdom, research into human ectogenesis is controlled by the Human Fertilisation and Embryology Bill (1990). This bill passed into law the recommendations of the so-called Warnock Committee. That committee, in 1984, made the following comments about ectogenesis as part of its report:

> It has been suggested that in the long term further development of current techniques could result in the maintenance of developing embryos in an artificial environment (ectogenesis) for progressively longer periods with the ultimate aim of creating a child entirely *in vitro* …
> We appreciate why the possibility of such a technique arouses so much anxiety. There are however two points to make about this. First, such developments are well into the future, certainly beyond the time horizon within which this Inquiry feels it can predict. Secondly, our recommendation is that the growing of a human embryo *in vitro* beyond fourteen days should be a criminal offence.[29]

This recommendation of the *Warnock Report* was ratified by the passing of the aforementioned Human Fertilisation and Embryology Bill (1990), clause 11 of which makes experimentation on human embryos more than 14 days old a criminal offence. Given the attitude of the *Warnock Report* to the prospect of ectogenesis, this clause is clearly aimed at preventing research into complete ectogenesis.

---

[29] Mary Warnock, *A Question of Life: The Warnock Report on Human Fertilisation and Embryology*, (Oxford: Basil Blackwell, 1985), pp. 71–2.

Current Laws: United States

As I stated earlier, I will not be reviewing the laws that relate to ectogenetic research in all 50 states. However, I would like to briefly mention the legal situation with regard to federal funding for ectogenetic research. Research into incomplete ectogenesis is permitted, and there is no problem in utilising federal funding for this type of research. However, research into complete ectogenesis, while not actually contrary to federal law, does run into some funding problems. At present in the United States, there is a congressional ban on the use of federal funding for foetal and embryo research. This ban obviously affects research into complete ectogenesis. The ban is also very broad ranging – if even a single piece of equipment in the laboratory has been purchased using federal funding, then the research is illegal. However, there are states where research into complete ectogenesis might be permitted, providing that the research used exclusively private funding.

Animal Research

The use of animals in research is almost universally accepted in the scientific community. Research involving animals is subject to far less stringent controls than research involving human subjects, and animals are frequently used in research in situations where research using human subjects would not be permitted. The case of embryonic and foetal research is no different. Where guidelines exist to control the use of animals in experiments, these guidelines generally only deal with the need to ensure that the suffering of experimental subjects is kept to a minimum. This is especially true for research involving animal embryos and foetuses. For example, the NHMRC in Australia prepared the Australian Code of Practice for the care and use of animals for scientific purposes. The sections in this code concerned with foetal experimentation on animals (3.3.65-8), deal only with the need for adequate pain relief for foetuses during surgery or other noxious experimentation on their mothers. Destructive experiments on animal embryos and foetuses are considered to be quite permissible, provided that adequate pain relief is provided in cases where it is plausible to think that the animal may suffer.

Given these facts, it is likely that research towards complete ectogenesis would begin on animals. I have been unable to find any laws, regulations or guidelines in any jurisdiction anywhere in the world that would prevent research aimed at complete ectogenesis, provided that this research used animal rather than human embryos.

Conclusions

This brief examination shows the current legal status of ectogenetic research fairly clearly. Research into incomplete ectogenesis is within the law in all the jurisdictions that I have examined. Research into complete ectogenesis in humans is generally outside the law, and in most other jurisdictions where such research is strictly legal, it would not be eligible for federal funding. However, animal research towards complete ectogenesis does not face the same restrictions, and may be both legal and eligible for federal funding in all jurisdictions.

Chapter 3

Theoretical Foundations

It is a truth about the human world that people disagree about almost everything. If one person asserts that *A* is true, then there will be someone else who asserts that *A* is not true. This disagreement reaches into virtually every aspect of human affairs, and in few fields is this disagreement as obvious as it is in ethics. There is no theory of ethics that has found universal agreement; no set of rules or principles for deciding ethical disputes that everyone can agree to. Yet in order to examine the ethical implications of something, it is obvious that some sort of theoretical basis will be required. My topic is, of course, no exception. I cannot examine the ethical implications of ectogenesis without setting out the principles upon which I will base the examination. Thus this chapter is an attempt to lay out what I believe to be the most defensible ethical foundations for an investigation of the ethical implications of human ectogenesis.

I should be clear from the very start as to what I will and will not do. It is not my intention to engage in lengthy debate about the relative merits of the major types of ethical theory, nor is it my intention to exhaustively catalogue the problems of individual versions of these theories. Rather, I will lay out the main tenets of the major types of ethical theory, and seek some common threads that might be utilised in later discussion. For while there can be striking differences in what actions the theories prescribe in extreme cases, such as in cases where a person must kill one in order to save five, the different theories do tend to agree on most everyday cases. This suggests that there must be some important common themes among the theories. It is my intention, as far as possible, to make use of these common themes in the discussion of the implications of ectogenesis that follows.

The three main classes of ethical theory that I wish to consider in this discussion are Consequentialist theories (primarily Utilitarianism), Kantian (deontological) and rights-based theories, and Virtue (Neo-Aristotelian) theories. What might the three main types of ethical theory say about the possibility of ectogenesis? Would a Virtue theorist see things differently from a Consequentialist, and would they see the situation differently from a Kantian?

Consequentialist Theories [1]

Consequentialist ethical theories focus on the outcomes of actions rather than the intentions behind the action or the character of the action itself. Actions are judged as right or wrong only in regard to the consequences that follow from the action. No action or action type is right or wrong in and of itself, it is only made right or wrong by the good or bad consequences that it produces. Different forms of consequentialism define what is good in different ways. For example, the most well known form of consequentialism, classical utilitarianism, defines the good as utility: maximising pleasure and minimising pain. A more sophisticated version of utilitarianism is preference utilitarianism, which aims to maximise the satisfaction of preferences of morally significant beings. This version has gained wide acceptance among contemporary utilitarians, and has important features in common with other major theories that I will examine.

There are two main things that all consequentialist theories have in common. The first idea common to all consequentialist theories is that rightness and wrongness are defined solely in terms of the consequences of actions; that is, by the goodness or badness of states of affairs that one brings about. Thus, acts are considered to be right or wrong not intrinsically, but by virtue of their consequences. An act that brings about the best available consequences is a right act; if it does not, then it is a wrong act. Thus an act could be the right thing to do in one situation, and the wrong thing to do in another. However, the important fact to note here is that all actions will be considered to be right or wrong only by virtue of their consequences; the action is never intrinsically right or wrong, and the intentions of the agent are intrinsically unimportant. The only thing that is important is maximising whatever good is prescribed by the theory.

The second aspect common to all consequentialist theories is that they have a monistic theory of value. Thus for a classical utilitarian, for example, the only thing that is intrinsically good is utility; promoting pleasure and avoiding pain. All other apparent goods, such as friendship, love, or learning, are instrumental goods, in that such goods increase overall utility. The goodness of these other things is explained entirely in terms of their contribution to maximising utility. In theory virtually anything could serve as 'the good' that a particular brand of consequentialism seeks to maximise, but in practice some goods are more plausible than others. While a consequentialist theory that sought to maximise human suffering is theoretically possible, in practice such a theory would have few (if any) supporters.

One of the major advantages of consequentialist theories is their simplicity. The goal of any piece of moral decision-making is clear; promotion of utility whether this is seen in terms of pleasure and minimisation of suffering, or preference satisfaction - so the questions for decision makers are largely pragmatic, directed to means-end considerations. Since such theories reduce moral decision-making to a

[1] This discussion draws on Philip Pettit, 'Consequentialism', and Robert E. Goodin, 'Utility and the Good', both in Peter Singer (ed.), *A Companion to Ethics*, (Oxford: Basil Blackwell, 1993).

single factor (promotion of utility for example), consequentialist theories are commonly used for determining the correct action in large-scale decisions, such as the allocation of medical resources. As long as the alternatives can be assessed in terms of a single factor, consequentialist theories will always be able to provide an answer as to what is the right thing to do.

Take the allocation of medical resources as an example. Suppose I need to decide the right way to spend the money that I have available, and have to choose between allocating that money to hip-replacement operations, or to kidney transplant operations. If I can evaluate the competing options by reference to a single value/measure which I am seeking to promote, then a consequentialist theory will tell me what the right way to spend the money is. In allocation of medical resources, the usual means of comparison is the Quality Adjusted Life Year, or QALY, which measures the benefits of treatment in terms of the number of years of life gained by the treatment, and the quality of life gained.[2] If allocating this money to kidney transplants will produce more QALYs than allocating the money to hip-replacements, then the right thing to do would be to allocate the money to kidney transplants. The fact that the good can be reduced to a single factor, in this case maximisation of QALYs, makes the decision simple.

There are two main criticisms of consequentialist theories. The first criticism is that many decisions involve situations that are either not easily reducible to a single factor or where the consequences are difficult to calculate. The second criticism is that because such theories do not give sufficient weight to the needs of individuals, they seem to allow, and even promote, unspeakable acts in certain situations.

Let me give an example of the first problem.[3] Suppose that I want to go to a 'Freedom from Hunger' rally, and the only way that I can get there is to drive my car. On the one hand I know that such rallies are important, and that my attendance will have some effect, albeit a small one, on world famine relief. On the other hand, I know that driving my car will have an effect, albeit a small one, on global environmental change. A situation like this seems to involve consequences of two sorts that are difficult, though perhaps not impossible, to compare, (famine relief and global change) and are also difficult to accurately calculate.

The second problem with consequentialist theories can also be illustrated. Since such theories are only concerned with overall consequences, and not with the consequences to particular individuals, this seems to suggest that such theories would allow, and even encourage, some situations that seem, to common sense morality, to be wrong. For example, if the best consequences for a particular

---

[2] For a discussion of the role of QALYs in health care see John Cubbon, 'The Principle of QALY Maximisation as the Basis for Allocating Health Care Resources', *Journal of Medical Ethics*, 17 (1991), pp. 181–4. For a criticism of the use of QALYs see John Harris, 'Unprincipled QALYs: A Response to Cubbon', *Journal of Medical Ethics*, 17 (1991), pp. 185–8.

[3] Drawn from an example by Dale Jamieson, 'When Utilitarians Should Be Virtue Theorists: The Case of Global Environmental Change', Presented at the International Conference on Applied Ethics, Hong Kong, December 1999.

society would flow from allowing slavery, then it would be wrong to prohibit slavery in that society. Most consequentialists would argue that such a case would be extremely unlikely, but must admit that it is still possible that slavery might be the right thing in some societies at some times. Some consequentialist theorists attempt to get around this problem by recognising a respect for the autonomy of persons as an important consideration in moral decision-making.[4] For example, preference utilitarians give strong weight to considerations of autonomy, since most people have very strong preferences that they (and not anyone else) control their lives.[5] These strong preferences would almost certainly rule out the permissibility of slavery in any society.

An extension of the second problem is the fact that consequentialism makes nothing unthinkable, for even the most horrifying acts might, in some circumstances, produce the best consequences, and thus be morally required. To illustrate this point further, let us consider an extreme example. Let us suppose that a pair of terrorists have planted an atomic bomb in the middle of a large city, and that the only way to find the bomb before it detonates (killing millions of people) is to torture the children of these terrorists, thus forcing the terrorists to reveal the location of the bomb. In this case, torturing the terrorist's children will bring about the best consequences, since it will save millions of lives. So for a consequentialist, torturing the terrorist's children is the right thing to do – not merely permissible, but actually required. This is the case even if the torturer is doing the torturing because he/she enjoys it, rather than for any higher motive, such as saving the innocent lives.

Many people would wish to say that such acts are never the right thing to do, or that at the very least such actions should be seen as choosing the lesser of two evils and are thus morally regrettable, a conclusion that a consequentialist would reject. This leads such people to reject consequentialism, and seek a theory that does contain prohibitions against acts such as these.

Kantian Theories [6]

These theories focus on universal principles that govern an agent's *action,* rather than on principles that govern the *outcome* of actions. What is good or bad, right or wrong, is defined by reference to a set of duties which it is claimed we owe to each other, rather than being defined by consequences. While there are many different ways of formulating this set of duties, one thing that all of these theories have in common is the idea that it is in following these duties that a person does the right

---

[4] See Jonathon Glover, *Causing Death and Saving Lives*, (Harmondsworth: Penguin, 1977), pp. 74–85.
[5] See Peter Singer, *Practical Ethics,* 2nd ed., (Cambridge: Cambridge Unievrsity, 1993), pp. 99–101.
[6] This discussion draws on Onora O'Neill, 'Kantian Ethics'; Brenda Almond, 'Rights'; and Nancy (Ann) Davis, 'Contemporary Deontology' all in Peter Singer (ed.), *A Companion to Ethics*, (Oxford: Basil Blackwell, 1993).

thing, even if this leads to worse consequences than could be achieved by breaking the rules. Kant, often seen as the father of theories of this type, suggested that people should only act by rules that could be universalised.[7] For example, one could not universalise the idea that people ought to lie, since this would bring an end to the practices of communication upon which lying depends, thus one should always tell the truth. Lying is wrong not because of any perceived bad consequences, but because the practice could not be universalised. The second overriding consideration in creating these universal rules is that they should be formulated in such a way that they treat all persons as ends in themselves. In the words of Kant, 'act so that you treat humanity, whether in your own person or in that of another, always as an end and never as a means only'.[8] Such a principle demands that people act in such a way that they leave other people free to act, and effectively rules out violations of another person's liberty. Thus while most consequentialist theories see individuals as mere receptacles of utility, interchangeable in most respects, this is not the case with deontological theories, which see respect for the autonomy of agents as a fundamental value.

Perhaps the most influential modern deontological theories are explicitly rights-based theories.[9] According to these theories, all moral agents have certain rights, which should be respected by all other moral agents. These rights include such things as the right to life, the right to liberty, the right to freedom of action and the right to own property. The theory of rights can be derived from a Kantian respect for persons; treating other moral agents as ends in themselves means respecting their rights.

Rights-based theories tend to give the individual priority over the community. Taking rights theories seriously means that the rights of a single individual cannot be traded off for the common good, even if this means that the overall community will suffer. In fact, the theory of rights can be seen as a means of protecting individuals against the desires of the community. For example, it would be impermissible to deliberately kill one person in order to save another five, since deliberately killing that one person would be a violation of their right to life. However, most rights-based theories recognise that not all rights are absolute, so it will be justifiable to violate the rights of people in some circumstances, usually when the more fundamental rights of another person would otherwise be violated. Rights are one of the most widely recognised moral concepts of our time, partly because of the formulation by the United Nations of the Universal Declaration of Human Rights in 1948. In has become quite common for people to talk about human rights violations, most often in other countries, but sometimes in their own country. The wide acceptance of rights talk is certainly one of the strengths of the theory.

---

[7] Immanuel Kant, *Foundations of the Metaphysics of Morals*, trans. L. W. Beck (New York, Macmillan, 1990), p. 38.
[8] *Foundations of the Metaphysics of Morals*, p. 46.
[9] Respect for the rights of persons is also an important part of some consequentialist theories. See for example Glover, *Causing Death and Saving Lives*, pp. 74–85.

Most deontological theories are framed in the form of negative duties; they primarily state what should not be done, rather than what should be done. The non-religious parts of the biblical ten commandments for example, form a set of deontological restraints, forbidding murder, theft, lying and adultery.[10] Kantian formulations also tend to end up as constraints on actions, and most rights also take the form of prohibitions. What this means in practice is that deontological theories are less restrictive than consequentialist theories. Consequentialist theories, being maximising theories, have only two classes of action; right or wrong (see the previous section on consequentialist theories). But deontological theories, which are not maximising theories, have three classes of action; impermissible, permissible, and obligatory.

Since most deontological rules are formulated as negative duties, the most basic class of actions for these types of theories are those that are impermissible. The obligatory actions are an extension of the impermissible actions, in that obligatory actions are those that are impermissible to omit.[11] The majority of actions will not fall into the category of the impermissible or the obligatory, and so will be deemed permissible. As Charles Fried expresses the point 'after having avoided wrong and doing one's duty, an infinity of choices is left to be made'.[12]

Because deontological theories focus on universal rules, they are, like consequentialist theories, useful for making large-scale decisions. One simply applies the universal rule to every individual in the community, or to the policy being proposed, to see if it meets the constraints of respect for the rights of others. But the one thing that all deontological theories (including rights-based theories) have in common is that actions are judged as right or wrong on the basis of whether the appropriate rule allows or forbids them, not on their consequences. So to return to the terrorist case, if the particular version of deontology that you were following forbade torture (as virtually every deontological theory does) then it would be wrong to torture the terrorist's children. This would be the case even if millions of people would die if the terrorist's children were not tortured, and even if the torturer hated what they were doing, and only had the intention of saving the millions of lives. A decision to torture the terrorist's children might be seen as choosing the lesser of two evils, but would still involve doing something seriously wrong.

Virtue Theories[13]

Virtue theories focus on the character of the agent, rather than on principles of action or the consequences of an action. Virtue theories generally define what is

---

[10] Exodus 20: 13–16.

[11] See Davis, 'Contemporary Deontology', p. 209.

[12] *Right and Wrong*, (Cambridge MA: Harvard University, 1978), p. 13.

[13] This discussion draws on Greg Pence, 'Virtue Theory', in Peter Singer (ed.), *A Companion to Ethics*, (Oxford: Basil Blackwell, 1993) and on Justin Oakley, 'Varieties of Virtue Ethics', *Ratio* 9 (1996), pp. 128–52.

good in terms of what is required for human flourishing, and suggest that a good person will cultivate those virtues that are necessary to allow the agent to flourish. The virtues required will include such things as honesty, courage, fidelity, and charity. Thus virtue ethics emphasises the moral character of the agent, rather than examining the action. Virtue theories claim that an action is right if and only if it is what a perfectly virtuous agent would do in the circumstances. The varieties of virtue ethics generally diverge around how the 'perfectly virtuous agent' is to be defined. However, if the ideal virtuous agent is to be defined in fairly general terms, then it will be no surprise if both deontological and consequentialist considerations contribute to the definition. Thus in the terrorist case, a virtue ethicist would suggest that torture is generally wrong in principle, not because of any perceived bad consequences but because this is the sort of act that a virtuous person would not be involved in. But in this particular situation it might be considered the right thing to do to torture the terrorist's children, because of the horrendous consequences of not doing so. In other words, the virtuous person would normally not countenance torture, but in these circumstances they might well concede that the right (or perhaps the least wrong) thing to do in these unusual circumstances would be to torture the terrorist's children.

While there is disagreement about how the virtuous agent is to be defined, there are some characteristics that can be assumed to hold true for all conceptions of the virtuous agent. Benevolence seems like a good example here, as do courage, wisdom, honesty, and respect for other agents. In this aspect of ethics at least, a virtue theorist seems to share some similarities with a deontologist, for both theories would seem to share a respect for persons as ends in themselves.

Because virtue theories focus on individuals, and not on general principles or consequences, they tend to make for more complicated assessments of what is right and wrong in a particular case. For example, the same kind of act could well be right for one person and wrong for another, depending upon the character of the agent involved, and the individual circumstances of the case. This means that virtue theories are highly sensitive to particular circumstances, which makes them rather less than useful in making large-scale decisions. A consequentialist would simply reduce a large-scale decision to a single variable, such as a QALY. A deontologist would see if the large-scale decision breached any particular rules. But a virtue theorist would need to know all the facts of the particular cases, and the characters of the agents involved, before they would be able to determine what was the right thing and wrong thing to do in that case. Thus virtue theory would not say that abortion (for example) is always right, or always wrong, but rather would suggest that abortion is right or wrong depending upon the circumstances of the case. Such a determination is not particularly helpful in determining whether abortion should be legal.

Seeking Common Ground

What common threads can be drawn from these different theories that would allow an examination of the ethical implications of a new technology like ectogenesis?

The most obvious area of common ground seems to be acknowledgment of the moral importance of respect for the autonomy of persons. This Kantian notion seems an essential part of deontological theories, including theories of rights, it is a concept that would be important to the virtuous person, and is also important to several influential versions of consequentialism (notably preference utilitarianism). Given its wide acceptance as a general principle, I would suggest that it is reasonable to begin with an examination of the nature of autonomy, and discussion of what a right to autonomy might entail.

So what is autonomy? Put simply, acting autonomously means acting freely and basing those free actions on rational principles. Thus a right to autonomy is a right to live one's own life without the unwanted interference of others. A violation of the right to autonomy involves either an interference in a person's ability to control significant parts of their own life or a lack of respect for a person's ability to control their own life. Thus a violation of the right to autonomy does not have to involve actual interference in the decisions of another person, it can simply be a lack of respect for their ability to make decisions, or a lack of respect for the decisions that they eventually make. For example, if I continually make decisions for another person, then I am showing a lack of respect for their right to autonomy. This would still be the case even if it could be shown that the decisions that I have made were in the best interests of the person whose autonomy I was violating.

It should be noted that not all creatures have autonomy, and that not all creatures can plausibly be seen as having a right to autonomy. There are certain attributes that are necessary for a creature to even have the possibility of autonomy, and even creatures that possess all of these features may not ever exercise autonomy.

So what features are necessary for a creature to possess autonomy? Essentially, what is required are those features which are commonly said to be required for one to be a 'person' in the philosophical sense of the term. Mary Anne Warren suggests that they include the following: Consciousness (in particular the capacity to feel pain), Reasoning, Self-Motivated Activity, The Capacity to Communicate, and The Presence of Self-Awareness.[14] A creature that is lacking all of these attributes is clearly not a candidate for autonomy, while a creature that possesses all of these attributes seems to have an unequivocal right to autonomy. Another way of defining the necessary attributes for autonomy is to look at the preferences of the creature involved. A being that acts only on immediate preferences, or on instinct, such as a lizard or a snake, does not seem to be a candidate for autonomy. However, a creature that has future-oriented preferences, such as a normal adult human being, does seem to be a candidate for autonomy.

To summarise, I will give some examples of creatures that would, and would not, qualify as candidates for autonomy. Most living creatures do not seem to be candidates for autonomy, since they do not seem to possess future-oriented desires. The only likely exceptions to this are mammals, especially the higher mammals such as primates, whales and dolphins, dogs and elephants. However, even within

---

[14] From Mary Anne Warren, 'On the Moral and Legal Status of Abortion', in R. Wasserstrom (ed.), *Today's Moral Problems*, (New York: MacMillan, 1975), p. 130.

these groups of mammals, there are some individuals that do not seem to possess the necessary attributes to be considered to be autonomous. The foetuses of all of these types of animals, for example, do not seem to possess any of the five attributes mentioned by Warren. Corpses of these species obviously do not possess the necessary features, and neither do severely brain-damaged individuals of any of these species.

Autonomy and Derivative Rights

Having briefly defined autonomy in this way, it is necessary to examine what other rights might plausibly be derived from the right to autonomy, especially, given the topic of this thesis, in regard to reproduction. The first right that can be derived from the right to autonomy is the right to life. Someone who kills an autonomous individual, without that individual's consent, has clearly violated that person's right to autonomy. The right to life is obviously extremely important – if you are dead then you certainly can't assert your right to autonomy. However, it can be argued that this right (as is the case with most rights derived from the right to autonomy) is essentially negative – that it is a right to not be unjustly killed, but that it does not allow a person to insist on being provided everything that they need to sustain their life. This point has been argued by Judith Jarvis Thomson in her famous paper 'A Defence of Abortion',[15] and is a point to which I will return in a later chapter.

Apart from the right to life, are there other rights that can be derived from the right to autonomy? Most importantly for the purposes of this current discussion, is it possible to derive a right to reproduce from the right to autonomy? I think that the right to reproduce can be derived from the right to autonomy in the following way. I have suggested that autonomy is the ability to plan for one's future, to make decisions regarding one's own life, and to freely implement those decisions. For very many people, reproduction and parenting is a central part of their life plan. It may well be the most meaningful part of their lives, possibly because it is seen as having religious significance, or as an expression of a couple's love. Inability to reproduce, for example through infertility, is often experienced as a great loss. Now if autonomy is the ability to make and implement decisions about one's own life, and if reproduction is a central part of many people's life plan, then it would seem that reproduction is an expression of autonomy, and that a right to autonomy entails a right to make one's own reproductive choices. In other words, a right to autonomy entails a right to reproduce.[16]

If the right to reproduce is derived from the right to autonomy, is the right to reproduce a purely negative right, or is it a positive right? In other words, is it simply a right to not be prevented from having children, or does it imply some

---

[15] Judith Jarvis Thomson, 'A Defence of Abortion', in R. Wasserstrom (ed.), *Today's Moral Problems*, (New York: MacMillan, 1975), pp. 104–19.
[16] For a more detailed exposition of this position see John Robertson, *Children of Choice*, (Princeton: Princeton University, 1994).

positive duties for others? It certainly appears that the right to reproduce is at the very least a right not to have others interfere in one's reproductive decisions – what John Robertson terms procreative liberty.[17] This would include both the right to have children, and the right to not have children. However, there does not seem to be an obvious obligation for anyone else to assist a person in exercising the right to reproduce, though of course they could assist if they wished to. For example, if a particular man wished to have children, he could not coerce his choice of female partner to get her to assist him in having children. She could choose to assist him in having children (by becoming pregnant with his child) or she could refuse to assist, but he has no right to coerce her. Equally, if she chooses to assist him, then no one else would have the right to prevent them from attempting to have children, unless the rights of others are going to be violated in a serious way.[18]

Thus it would seem that the right to reproduce is merely a negative right, and that the general theory of rights based on autonomy has little to say about most reproductive choices, other than to suggest that they are generally permissible. But this does not seem to really be an adequate response when we wish to make large-scale decisions about the morality of particular options in regard to reproduction. For example, we might ask questions like 'Should we allow the use of abortiofacients like RU486? Should we allow commercial surrogacy arrangements to take place? Should we allow the manipulation of embryos with the aim of allowing parents to choose the sex of their baby?' All of these questions do not seem to be adequately answered by a simple rights-based framework that merely suggests that they may be permissible. In order to make adequate moral decisions about such cases, I would suggest that we need to move beyond a straight forward rights-based framework, and look at the possible consequences of each option in such cases.

When discussing public policy, it seems inadequate to merely suggest that something may be 'permissible'. Merely discussing whether people's autonomy might be harmed or enhanced by allowing a particular technology to become available seems an insufficient response. At the very least we expect that governments will assess likely demands on the public purse from allowing a new technology to be developed, and then compare those likely demands with other existing demands when deciding on the disposition of public funds. Given that public funds are always a limited resource, cases like this seem to require an examination of the likely consequences as well. We also expect governments to take into consideration the beliefs and desires of members of society when deciding upon a legislative framework that might affect a new technology, and to consider the likely consequences for other members of society when doing so. If developing a particular technique, like ectogenesis for example, will bring about good consequences, then it should be done. If it will bring about bad consequences,

---

[17] *Ibid.*

[18] There may be some cases where we think that someone does not have a right to reproduce, and thus that they should be prevented from reproducing. An example of this might be when we can be sure that any children produced will be severely disabled. The possibility of such cases does not refute the general suggestion that generally reproduction is permissible, as opposed to being mandatory or impermissible.

then it should not be done. When rights-based theories cannot do any more than to suggest that something is permissible, and more guidance is required on that subject, then the rights-based approach must be broadened to include an analysis of consequences. If the consequences of allowing or facilitating a *prima facie* 'permissible' procedure will be dire, then it would seem that the right thing to do is not to allow the procedure. If the consequences will be good, then the procedure should be allowed. Introducing consequences in this way moves us from a simple rights-based theory to a more sophisticated rights/consequences theory. When rights give no clear answers, then consequences must be taken into account if we are to make truly informed ethical decisions. However, I would agree with John Robertson in suggesting that given the importance of autonomy, the basic presumption should be in favour of procreative liberty,[19] since more choice will generally allow more room for freedom, and thus the expression of autonomy. Thus unless there is clear evidence that the consequences of allowing a particular procedure will be bad, the procedure should be allowed.

Procreative Liberty and Ectogenesis

Given the presumption of procreative liberty, there is no need for any great argument in favour of developing any new reproductive technology, for the onus is on the opponents of the technology to show that there are weighty objections against its development and use. Thus I do not think that there is any need for me to present a detailed argument in favour of the development of ectogenesis. It is sufficient to merely point out the various ways in which such an argument might be formulated, and then move on to consider the objections that might be presented.

In Chapter 5 of their book *The Reproduction Revolution,*[20] Peter Singer and Deane Wells list five arguments that might be made in favour of pursuing ectogenetic research.[21] In addition to the arguments presented by Singer and Wells, Laura Purdy presents a feminist argument in favour of the development of ectogenesis.[22] It is quite possible that any one of these arguments would, given the assumption of procreative liberty, be strong enough to justify the development of ectogenesis. Since I will be considering many of these arguments in detail in later chapters, I will do no more than sketch out the bones of each of the arguments

---

[19] Robertson, *Children of Choice*, p. 16.

[20] Peter Singer and Deane Wells, *The Reproduction Revolution: New Ways of Making Babies*, (Oxford: Oxford University, 1984). Revised North American edition published as *Making Babies: The New Science and Ethics of Conception*, (New York: Scribners, 1985). The relevant chapter is Chapter 5 and is found at pp. 131–149 in the Oxford edition, pp. 116–34 in the Scribners edition.

[21] Singer and Wells do not actually give each of these arguments names, but they are named by David V. James, in his reply to this chapter. See 'Ectogenesis: A Reply to Singer and Wells', *Bioethics*, 1 (1987), pp. 80–99.

[22] In 'The Morality of New Reproductive Technologies', in *Reproducing Persons*, (Ithaca: Cornell University, 1996).

here, as that is all that is necessary to show that there is a *prima facie* case for the development of ectogenesis.

Possibly the most interesting of Singer and Wells' arguments is the abortion reconciliation argument. They suggest that the development of ectogenesis might make it possible for the wishes of both anti-abortionist 'right-to-lifers' and pro-abortionist 'right-to-choosers' to be fulfilled. If ectogenesis became possible, it might then be possible to remove an unwanted foetus from the womb of the undesiring mother without ending its life, thus removing one of the main objections to abortion. As Singer and Wells point out 'it is only our inability to keep early foetuses alive that makes abortion synonymous with the violation of any right to life which the foetus may have.'[23]

Another argument presented by Singer and Wells is the Better Surrogacy argument. In any society there will always be some women who are incapable of pregnancy, perhaps because they have had a hysterectomy, or because they have a medical condition that makes pregnancy too dangerous. For women in this position who wish to have children there are two alternatives; adoption or surrogacy. If these women wish to raise a child that is genetically related to them, then there is only one alternative; surrogacy. But surrogacy is considered to be problematic for various reasons, such as the possibility that it exploits women, or that it might lead to the commodification of children. All of these factors combined seem to form quite a strong case for the development of ectogenesis, which would avoid most, if not all of these problems.

Singer and Wells also suggest that a strong argument for pursuing ectogenetic research could be advanced on the basis that it would enable partial ectogenesis for transplant. Modern medicine uses tissue and organ transplants in a large number of ways, and that number is continually increasing. But there is always a shortage of suitable organs for transplant purposes. Ectogenetic technology would allow foetuses to be developed specifically for the purpose of producing organs for the purposes of transplant, thus eliminating the problem of a lack of available organs.

In addition to these arguments, Singer and Wells also mention two arguments in favour of the development of ectogenesis that were suggested by the feminist writer Shulamith Firestone.[24] She suggested that ectogenesis ought to be developed because it would lead to real equality between the sexes, by allowing the reproductive labour to be divided equally between members of the family. She also suggested that ectogenesis would produce better parents, since mothers would no longer feel the possessiveness of their children that is caused by having to undergo the pain of labour.

Laura Purdy's argument for developing ectogenesis concentrates on the problems with current reproduction.[25] Medically speaking, pregnancy is, in some cases, undeniably risky. Complications associated with childbirth are one of the leading causes of death in women of child-bearing age.[26] Other medical problems

---

[23] Singer and Wells, *Reproduction Revolution*, p. 135.
[24] See *The Dialectic of Sex*, (New York: Bantam, 1971).
[25] 'The Morality of New Reproductive Technologies'.
[26] *Ibid.*, p. 178.

can be exacerbated by pregnancy, such as kidney disease, diabetes, liver disease, and cardiac problems.[27] Even for otherwise healthy women, pregnancy is a cause of nausea, cramps, haemorrhoids, heartburn, varicose veins and nosebleeds.[28] Given the problems that pregnancy can cause, it seems reasonable to attempt to develop an alternative, such as ectogenesis, even if this alternative was only to be used in cases where pregnancy was likely to cause risk of serious harm to the mother.

Given all of these arguments in favour of developing ectogenesis, and the assumption of the primacy of procreative liberty, there does seem to be a *prima facie* case for developing this technology. Whether there exist objections to the technology that are serious enough to preclude its development is the topic of the next chapter.

[27] *Ibid.*, pp. 178–9.
[28] *Ibid.*, p. 179.

Chapter 4

Objections to Ectogenesis

A number of objections might be raised to the possibility of ectogenesis. I wish, in this chapter to consider a number of these objections, and see if they are serious enough to warrant the bans on ectogenesis that currently exist in a number of jurisdictions. Some of the objections are rather familiar, since they have been raised against many forms of reproductive technology. I will discuss them since they have at times been directed specifically at ectogenesis. As far as other general objections go, I will only concentrate on those objections that seem to have extra significance to ectogenesis. Thus there are six particular objections that I wish to examine in this chapter. One, the suggestion that we should concentrate on adoption as a means of providing children to the infertile, rather than developing and using sophisticated reproductive technology. Two, the suggestion that it would be a poor use of resources to spend time and money on developing reproductive technologies like ectogenesis. Three, the possible harms to the child born through ectogenesis. Four, the argument that ectogenesis is 'unnatural' or 'playing God'. Five, the suggestion that the development of ectogenesis brings us one step closer to the famous dystopian vision of the future presented by Aldous Huxley in *Brave New World*.[1] Six, feminist objections to the development of ectogenesis.

The Better Surrogacy Argument

In *The Reproduction Revolution*,[2] Peter Singer and Deane Wells suggest that there are medical grounds for developing ectogenesis. Specifically they suggest that ectogenesis might be utilised by women for whom pregnancy is either impossible, or too dangerous, but who wish to have a child that is genetically related to them. For example, a woman who has had a hysterectomy would obviously find it impossible to fall pregnant, and a woman who has extremely high blood pressure would find pregnancy extremely dangerous to her health. Singer and Wells point out the only current alternative for such women is surrogacy, which is considered problematic for various reasons, none of which need to be considered here. The

---

[1] First published in Great Britain by Chatto and Windus, 1932. Currently available with a new introduction by Aldous Huxley, and biographical details of the author in the Flamingo Modern Classics series, 1994.
[2] Peter Singer and Deane Wells, *The Reproduction Revolution: New Ways of Making Babies*, (Oxford: Oxford University, 1984), pp. 134–6.

only other possible option for these women would be adoption, which would provide these women with a child, but not one that is genetically related to them. Singer and Wells are quite succinct in presenting their case:

> The medical case for ectogenesis, then, would consist of the medical case for surrogate motherhood, coupled with the claim that ectogenesis should be chosen in preference to surrogacy.[3]

This argument has been dubbed 'The Better Surrogacy Argument' by David James,[4] and is interesting to us primarily because of the objections that he presents in opposing the development of ectogenesis. These objections, that adoption should be preferred to reproductive technology, and that resources should not be allocated to the development of such technology, are quite general, and have been applied to other types of reproductive technology in the past. Since these objections are so general, they can be considered without examining the argument of Singer and Wells in any detail. It is sufficient to merely note that there are arguments that could be mounted for the development of ectogenesis, and that these arguments amount to a *prima facie* case for its development. Given that assumption, let us proceed to examine James' objections, and to see how these objections might be dealt with.[5]

James'criticism of the development of ectogenesis is mainly due to the fact that he believes that strong government support would be required to maintain the programme of development, and he believes that this programme is not something that should be receiving that sort of support. There are two main reasons why he holds this view. First, he questions the motivations of those who seek to use reproductive technology to assist them in their attempts to have children, and suggests that these people should be steered towards adoption instead. Second, he questions whether treatment of infertility should receive any government funding at all, given the other programmes that also require funding.

The Adoption Objection

James assumes that some desires that people have are entitled to state support, because these desires express fundamental interests of persons. He also assumes that the desire of the childless to nurture is such a fundamental interest. James suggests that if the desire to have children is a legitimate desire, then the state should encourage people unable to fulfil this desire to adopt unwanted children, rather than supplying them with new children through ectogenesis (or indeed through any other reproductive technology). His suggestion is that if infertile

---

[3] *Ibid.*, p. 134.
[4] David V. James, 'Ectogenesis: A Reply to Singer and Wells', *Bioethics*, 1 (1987), pp. 80–99.
[5] An earlier version of this section has previously been published as 'A Surrogate for Surrogacy? – The Artificial Uterus', *Australian Journal of Professional and Applied Ethics*, 1 (1999), pp. 49–60.

couples wish only to have a child that is genetically related to them, then this is not an interest that the state should support, for he believes that such an interest is based on an erroneous understanding of the facts of heredity, and as such fails to take into account other alternatives, such as adoption.[6]

So let us consider James' adoption objection. James considers three possible ways that the fundamental desire to nurture might be construed.[7] First, he suggests that this desire might be a very general one, that includes tutoring children, or visiting the elderly in nursing homes. Obviously, if this is all that the fundamental interest consists in, then virtually anyone can fulfil this desire with little difficulty, and without sophisticated technology. A second narrower, but still plausible meaning might be 'to have (or to parent) children'.[8] Fulfilling this desire might require state support, but would not require technology as sophisticated as an artificial uterus, for a state supported programme of adoption would clearly be sufficient to fulfil this desire. The third meaning that James considers is 'to have children genetically related to oneself'.[9] This desire James considers at best non-fundamental, and at worst possibly even morally abhorrent, for he considers it to be based on false assumptions about the importance of genetic ties, possibly underscored by racial or other prejudices.

Of these three meanings, the first can be satisfied without any sophisticated technology, and the third does not look to James like a desire that the state should help to satisfy, so only the second would need to be dealt with. Ectogenesis would allow couples to satisfy their desire in this second meaning of the phrase. However, adoption would also allow couples to fulfil this desire. In addition, adoption has several social benefits that ectogenesis does not have; it enriches the lives of unwanted children, relieves society of the expense of their care, and promotes the goal of limiting population.[10] James argues that practices that have social benefits and allow individuals to fulfil fundamental interests are preferable to other practices that allow the fulfilment of fundamental interests without producing social benefits. Ectogenesis allows the fulfilment of fundamental interests, but it does not produce social benefits. Adoption allows both the fulfilment of fundamental interests and the production of social benefits, so adoption should be preferred to ectogenesis. James has also applied the 'adoption objection' to other reproductive technologies,[11] especially artificial insemination with donor sperm.

This argument has been attacked by Paul Lauritzen in his book, *Pursuing Parenthood.*[12] Lauritzen points out that 'even in a strictly utilitarian calculus, we must examine the costs as well as the benefits, ... and this James does not do'.[13]

---

[6] *Ibid.*
[7] James, 'Ectogenesis', p. 93.
[8] *Ibid.*
[9] *Ibid.*
[10] *Ibid.*
[11] See, for example, his 'Artificial Insemination: A Re–Examination', *Philosophy and Theology*, 2 (1988), pp. 305–26.
[12] *Pursuing Parenthood*, (Bloomington: Indiana University, 1993).
[13] *Ibid.*, p. 121.

Certainly adoption produces certain benefits that are not produced by reproductive technologies that also fulfil the same fundamental interests. But it may also have costs that are not shared with other solutions. So let us examine the problems with current adoption practices, and see if these costs might outweigh the benefits produced. If the costs do outweigh the benefits, then it would seem that reproductive technologies might be preferable to adoption, despite their apparent lack of subsidiary benefits.

Problems with Current Adoption Practices   The most obvious problem with current adoptions is the lack of children available for adoption. This lack of children has led to long waiting periods and more stringent screening tests for prospective adopting couples. James considers this problem to be of minor importance, and suggests that 'the proper reply to couples who object to the long wait required to adopt is that they should learn the virtue of patience'.[14] However, as Lauritzen points out, this reply fails to grasp the implications of this problem. Long waiting lists have forced a change in emphasis from domestic to international adoptions, and from public agencies to private adoptions. This change has brought with it a host of new problems.

The popular model of adoptions is that of a non-profit public agency. Counsellors and social workers talk to birth mothers and prospective parents, screen for psychological problems, conduct home studies, and at all times seek the best result for the prospective adopted child. Yet Lauritzen points out the fallacy of treating this as the paradigm case of adoption, in the USA at least, for by 1993 in the USA only 5 per cent of domestic adoptions were arranged by such a public agency.[15] 50 per cent of all domestic adoptions in the USA were arranged independently, usually by an attorney, and 45 per cent of adoptions were arranged by private agencies, many of whom exist solely for profit.[16] The situation for international adoptions is similar, with both private for-profit agencies and independent individuals organising the vast majority of international adoptions.

Surrogacy is often criticised for commodifying babies, and commercialising reproduction. But current adoption practices also seem to fall foul of the same objection. In the USA in 1993 the average cost of a private adoption was $12,000 (compared to the average cost of a public adoption of $1,000). When one considers that in the famous Baby M surrogacy case, William Stern paid $25,000 dollars to the surrogacy agency that hired Mary Beth Whitehead in the hope of producing a child that would carry half his genetic code, the difference between the two does not seem to be so very great. The cost of an international adoption is often even greater and the recent trend of internet adoptions only emphasises this problem. Anyone concerned about the commodification of children by reproductive technology should also be concerned about the same problems in the current practices of adoption. In fact, I would suggest that this is even more of a problem

---

[14] 'Ectogenesis', p. 94.
[15] *Pursuing Parenthood*, p. 124.
[16] *Ibid.*

than it might first appear, when it is remembered that adoption is not only more widely practiced than say, surrogacy, but is also far more widely accepted.

Even one of the comforting aspects of the practice of adoption, the giving of a loving home to an unwanted child, turns out to be essentially an illusion. The vast majority of mothers do not relinquish children for adoption because they want to, but rather because they are forced to through poverty. They are not unwilling to care for the child, they are simply financially unable. This is especially the case with international adoption. Virtually all the children adopted internationally come from economically or politically oppressed areas, and this very fact is often used to encourage people to adopt them, to 'give them a better life'. Probably only the orphans from these areas can really be classed as 'unwanted'. Even within the USA, one study found that 69 per cent of parents giving children up for adoption cited external pressures, including financial constraints, as the primary reason for surrender.[17] All of this suggests that the comforting idea of 'unwanted children' finding loving homes is false.

It is now also recognised that surrendering a child for adoption is a deeply traumatic experience, and that this trauma is long lived. The logic of this is clear when the semi-coerced nature of many adoptions is recognised. If a mother does not want to give up her child, but is forced to through poverty (probably even feeling that this is the best thing for the child), then long-term psychological problems for the mother are only to be expected. There are costs to adoption, not only benefits, and every adoption involves loss and pain. In the words of Barbara Katz Rothman 'For every pair of welcoming arms, there is a pair of empty arms. For every baby taken in, there is a baby given up'.[18] There also seem to be disturbing issues of class involved. Rothman suggests that children are a product, exported from poor countries to rich ones, from blacks to white, from the poor to the better off, and that adoption agencies are an efficient system for redistributing children from the poor to the middle class.[19] Adoption is often assumed to benefit all concerned, but the evidence suggests that it is a system that takes advantage of a vulnerable group to satisfy the 'fundamental desires' of a far more secure group. Quite simply, adoption generally benefits the adoptive parents at the expense of the surrendering parents, particularly the birth mothers.

A Re-examination of the Adoption Objection   So where does this leave James' adoption objection? Balanced against the social benefits of enriching the lives of unwanted children, relieving society of the expense of their care, and promoting the goal of limiting population, we have the social problems of commodification of children, psychological problems in the surrendering parents, and disturbing issues of class inequality. Given these problems, adoption hardly looks the glowing alternative to reproductive technology that James suggests.

---

[17] Eva Y. Deykin et al., 'The Postadoption Experience of Surrendering Parents', *American Journal of Orthopsychiatry*, 54 (1984), p. 273.
[18] *Recreating Motherhood: Ideology and Technology in a Patriarchal Society*, (New York: N.W. Norton, 1989), p. 126.
[19] *Ibid.*, p. 130.

However, it should be remembered that the ideal case of adoption, basically that of the public non-profit agency, may be generally preferable to the use of sophisticated technology. If the technology is expensive, perhaps that money might be better spent on improving the practice of adoption, so that all adoptions meet this ideal standard. Of course, this still would not solve the problem of the pain of loss for the surrendering mothers, nor would it solve the problem of poverty, the cause of the 'unwantedness' of so many babies. Such discussions of the allocation of scarce resources lead us neatly into James' second objection to ectogenesis.

The Resource Allocation Objection

David James' second major objection to ectogenesis is essentially a financial one. James believes that a large amount of government funding would be required to initiate and maintain an ectogenetic programme, and he questions whether this sort of programme, and even the treatment of infertility generally, should receive any government funding, given the other priorities of the health-care budget. Singer and Wells suggest that infertility is a medical problem, a disability, and the amount of funding given to treatment of this problem should be decided solely in terms of how severe a disability it is, and what priority the treatment of infertility should have in the light of other demands on medical resources.[20] They compare the treatment of infertility with psychiatric treatment aimed at overcoming stress or anxiety, reasoning that infertility is a cause of stress and anxiety for the infertile couple:

> We think it would be absurd for the public purse to pay for a psychiatrist to attempt to treat the depression and anxiety caused by infertility but not to pay for the treatment of infertility itself. The desire for children is, in many people, something very basic and cannot be overcome without great difficulty, if at all. There are obvious evolutionary reasons why this should be so. We consider that it is quite appropriate for an affluent society to spend public funds on assisting its citizens to satisfy this desire.[21]

There are several questions that need to be addressed here, to see if Singer and Wells are correct in suggesting that the public purse should pay for infertility services. First, are they correct in suggesting that infertility is a disability? Second, if it is a disability, should the sorts of services that Singer and Wells are discussing be considered treatments for that disability? Third, if this is a treatment for a disability, is relief of this disability a high enough priority, given other demands on the health budget, for public funding to be allocated to the treatment? Only if all of these questions are answered in the affirmative would it seem to be appropriate for the public purse to pay for a programme of ectogenesis.

So are Singer and Wells correct in suggesting that infertility is a disability? Despite the suggestions of some critics of reproductive technology,[22] I would

[20] *Reproduction Revolution*, pp. 63–8.
[21] *Ibid.*, p. 67.
[22] For example, see Leon Kass, 'Babies by Means of In Vitro Fertilisation: Unethical Experiments on the Unborn?', *New England Journal of Medicine*, 285 (1971), pp. 1174–9.

suggest that the answer to this question must be yes. Some people are unable to do things that a fully functional person can do. A blind person cannot see, a paraplegic cannot use their legs, an infertile person cannot beget children. All are disabilities. Granted infertility is an unusual disability, since it involves an inability only in collaboration with another person, but it is a disability nonetheless. In some cases it may even be the case that a couple is jointly infertile, though either partner on their own may be considered to be fertile – for some reason the man's sperm will not fertilise his partner's eggs, though they can be fertilised by other men's sperm, and her partner's sperm can fertilise other women's eggs. Certainly this is an extremely unusual disability as far as disabilities go, but it still remains a disability.

Given that infertility is a disability, can the use of ectogenesis be considered to be a treatment for the disability? Again, some critics of reproductive technology have suggested that *In Vitro* Fertilisation (IVF) and similar procedures, such as ectogenesis, are not treatments for infertility, since they do not solve the underlying problem. A woman with blocked fallopian tubes, who achieves pregnancy through IVF, will still have blocked fallopian tubes. This is undeniably true, but this does not mean that IVF and other reproductive technologies are not treatments for infertility. As Singer and Wells point out, glasses do not cure short-sightedness, insulin treatment does not cure diabetes, yet these are both recognised treatments. If IVF is a recognised treatment for infertility caused by blocked fallopian tubes, then surely ectogenesis would have to be recognised as a treatment for infertility caused by lack of a uterus.

So it seems that infertility is a disability, and that ectogenesis might be a treatment for that disability. Given this, there remains only one question to be answered; is relieving this disability a high enough priority, given other demands on the health budget, for public funding to be allocated to the treatment? This is a much more difficult question to answer, and really depends upon which particular set of priorities are assumed. Let me give three examples here.

In their paper 'The Allocation of Medical Resources',[23] Maureen Sheehan and Deane Wells argue that an ideal allocation of medical resources would find a place for reproductive technology. They suggest that there are seven levels of priority for medical care, and that reproductive technology would fall somewhere between levels three (relieving serious physical or psychological pain) and six (improving the quality of people's lives). If this is the case, then it would seem likely that affluent societies would want to spend public money in relieving such problems.

However, a different view is presented by Darren Shickle.[24] His discussion of public priorities for health care in the United Kingdom found that people generally rated treatment for infertility as a low priority, usually only above alternative medicine and cosmetic surgery (City and Hackney Health Authority Survey) or treatment for people aged 75 and over with life-threatening illnesses (Office of

---

[23] 'The Allocation of Medical Resources', in C.L. Buchanan & E.W. Prior (eds), *Medical Care and Markets*, (Sydney: Allen & Unwin, 1985), pp. 59–69.
[24] 'Public Preferences for Health Care: Prioritisation in the United Kingdom', *Bioethics*, 11 (1997), pp. 277–90.

Population Censuses and Surveys). Given this sort of priority, it is unlikely that public funds would be diverted to the treatment of infertility.

A third example of possible prioritisation comes from the Oregon Health Services Commission in the USA. In attempting to prioritise spending in the Medicaid programme, the Oregon Health Services Commission held many public discussions, meetings with health service professionals and so on, and produced many lists of health spending priorities. Their priority list of 1991 lists infertility treatment services as 15th out of 17 sub-categories. Again, given this sort of priority, it is unlikely that government funds would be allocated to the relief of infertility.

So it would seem that the question of whether government funding should be available to assist the infertile is dependent upon what sort of priority we allocate to treatment of infertility, and that there is no real agreement about the priority that should apply. Certainly it appears that relieving the problems of the infertile ranks higher than some other areas of health care that do currently receive government funding (such as certain types of cosmetic surgery) but that is not enough to establish that infertility treatment should receive government funding, for it might be the case that those areas of health care with a lower priority ought not to be funded now. Infertility treatment would clearly be a priority for government funding if the health budget was unlimited, but in the real world that is unlikely to ever be the case.

What about Singer and Wells' suggestion that 'it would be absurd for the public purse to pay for a psychiatrist to attempt to treat the depression and anxiety caused by infertility but not to pay for the treatment of infertility itself'?[25] This raises an interesting question, since psychiatric services rank considerably higher than infertility services on most (if not all) prioritisation listings. Generally speaking, we tend to think that prevention is better than cure, and that it is better to treat the cause of a problem rather than the symptoms. Knowing that infertility services are available might prevent depression and anxiety amongst the infertile in the community, and if these psychiatric problems were caused by infertility problems, then surely it would be better to treat the cause of the problem, the infertility, rather than the symptoms.

But it would certainly cause resentment, and no doubt other related problems, if the only people who received government assistance for infertility treatments were those who had developed psychiatric problems due to their infertility.

Fortunately, in the case of ectogenesis, I think that there is an answer. While infertility treatments generally may attract government funding, on the basis that they are generally reasonably cost effective, this is unlikely to be true of ectogenesis. If the cost of ectogenesis is anything like the cost of care for a premature infant, then the cost per treatment would probably be enormous. Ectogenesis would only be required by a small percentage of the infertile (those who are simply unable to carry a child). Given the enormous cost, and the relatively small benefit, I think that whatever the government's health care priorities may be, it is unlikely that an ectogenetic treatment programme would be

[25] *Reproduction Revolution*, p. 67.

seen as a cost-effective way of managing the infertility problems of the relatively small number of infertile couples who would require the treatment. This is especially true when the cost of research is also taken into account. Many medical research programmes have spin-off benefits to other areas of medical science, but this seems unlikely in the case of ectogenetic research, which appears to be something of a dead end. While it may be generally the case that treating the cause is better than treating the symptoms, this is probably not still the case when treating the cause is likely to cost literally millions of dollars more than treatment and relief of the symptoms.

Conclusions: General Arguments Against Reproductive Technology

So do the problems of surrogacy lead to an argument in favour of developing an artificial uterus as a treatment for infertility? I think that the answer is both yes and no. Yes, an artificial uterus would help women who are unable to carry a child. There are objections to this position, but most of the objections can be dealt with. However, the one objection that does seem insurmountable is the problem of cost. Given the enormous sums of money that would need to be invested in such a programme, and the small number of people who would benefit, I think that the weight of argument comes down against the implementation of such a programme, assuming that government funds were required, simply because there are far better ways that this money could be spent, and even better ways that this money could benefit the infertile. However, if a private source wanted to fund such research, then I can see no direct objection. While I think that there are many better ways that such money could be spent, I do not think that there is any direct argument that can be presented to suggest that the money should not be spent pursuing the research and development of ectogenesis.

Harms to the Ectogenetic Child

Another more specific objection that has been made to the use of many forms of reproductive technology is the suggestion that the use of this technology would cause harm to the child produced. The argument is that the results of the use of the new technology cannot be fully predicted, and so there is a risk that there will be unexpected results, such as the baby being born severely deformed. This argument has been applied to reproductive technologies such as IVF, and Artificial Insemination, but it does appear to have particular force when brought against ectogenesis. This is because the harm likely to be done to the child is assumed to be psychological, rather than physical. In order to understand the importance of this argument, I will take a moment to examine the arguments against IVF, since similar arguments are proposed against ectogenesis. This is important, since it is only by gaining an understanding of the arguments against IVF that we can see the extra weight that the argument for harm to the child has against ectogenesis.

When the idea of using IVF to treat human infertility was first suggested, there were howls of protest from those who believed that the risks to the child were too great to justify the procedure. For example, one obstetrician, John Marlow, suggested that 'the potential is there for serious anomalies should an unqualified scientist mishandle an embryo'.[26] Leon Kass argued against all forms of reproductive technology in suggesting that 'It doesn't matter how many times the baby is tested while in the mother's womb, they will never be certain the baby won't be born without defect'.[27] Max Perutz, a Nobel Prize winner and former colleague of Robert Edwards (one of the scientists who assisted in producing the first IVF baby, Louise Brown) suggested that:

> ... this is far too great a risk. Even if only a single abnormal baby is born and has to be kept alive as an invalid for the rest of its life, Dr Edwards would have a terrible guilt upon his shoulders. The idea that this might happen on a larger scale – a new thalidomide catastrophe – is horrifying.[28]

Daniel Callahan, one of the founders of the Hastings Center, argued that the first case of IVF was probably unethical,[29] since there was no guarantee that Louise Brown would be born normal, though he did suggest that after this first healthy birth it would be ethical to proceed with IVF.

These arguments all emphasise the negative aspects of the procedure, without reference to the acceptance of risk by those undergoing IVF. Respect for autonomy would suggest that if people wish to subject themselves to risk (assuming that they fully understand that risk[30]), then they should be allowed to do so, unless other rights will be violated, or the consequences for society will be disastrous. The question of whether other rights are being violated is one to which I will return later. The dire consequences for society in this case seem to be considerably overstated by those condemning IVF, since if the procedure produced a high number of abnormalities, it is unlikely that many people would opt to take the risk. This problem with these arguments is pointed out by Gregory Pence:

> What these critics seem to overlook is that no reasonable approach to life can avoid all risks. Moreover, they also demonstrate a psychologically normal but nevertheless

[26] John Marlow, quoted in *U.S. News and World Report*, August 7, 1978, p. 24.
[27] Leon Kass, 'The New Biology: What Price Relieving Man's Estate?' *Journal of the American Medical Association*, 174 (Nov. 19, 1971), pp. 779–88.
[28] Max Perutz, quoted in Patrick Steptoe and Robert Edwards, *A Matter of Life: The Story of a Medical Breakthrough*, (London: Morrow, 1980), p. 163.
[29] Daniel Callahan, *New York Times*, July 27, 1978, p. A16.
[30] That the risk needs to be fully understood is an important, and sometimes overlooked point. Since I am mainly interested in the harms to the potential child, this point is not one that I am really able to pursue at this point in time. However, a number of authors have written at length on the subject of whether the women involved in IVF (especially in its early years) really understood the potential risks of the procedure. For extensive discussions on this issue, see Gena Corea, *The Mother Machine*, (London: The Women's Press, 1985/1988) and Robyn Rowland, *Living Laboratories*, (Sydney: Pan, 1992).

illogical tendency to magnify the risk of a harmful but unlikely event. A highly unlikely result – even if that result is very bad – still represents a very small risk.[31]

The physical risks to children born of IVF were certainly not zero, but there was some evidence available that suggested that children born of IVF were at no greater risk of deformity than children born by normal unaided sexual reproduction. There was data from animal experiments involving several different species, which suggested that IVF did not produce deformed offspring. The transfer of embryos was widely and successfully used in commercial animal breeding, apparently without any higher rate of abnormalities. It appeared in other animals that embryos either grew normally, or they died.[32] This suggested that similar results could be expected in humans.

It has been suggested that the data on animal experiments was rather generously interpreted, and that there were significant risks to the child involved in the procedure of IVF. For example, Gena Corea points out that the vast majority of data on embryo transfer in animals involves embryos obtained through uterine flushing, not through IVF. She also notes that there were few records kept of the rate of abnormalities in animals, since most of the transfers took place in a commercial, rather than a scientific, setting.[33] Embryologist Richard Blandau also questioned the data, asking 'Who would be concerned over any deficiency in creative ability in a cow or sheep?'[34] However, even if the risk of deformities was increased, it seems absurd to suggest that this means the procedure should never be used. Many procedures carry increased risks over the alternatives, but they commonly have increased benefits as well. The oral contraceptive pill is certainly more of a medical risk than the alternative of condoms, but it does have other benefits. In the case of IVF, even if there does exist an increased risk of a deformed baby, the alternative for many couples would be to not have children at all. This unattractive alternative seems to make the increased risk worthwhile. We can now see, over 20 years down the track, that the fears that IVF would produce abnormal babies have certainly been laid to rest, and there are now tens of thousands of perfectly normal IVF children scattered throughout the world.

Another suggestion that was made when IVF first came to prominence was that the children of IVF would be psychologically harmed, by being conceived in such an unusual way. For example, Father Laurence Fitzgerald suggested that:

With all the publicity that has surrounded *in vitro* births, it is hard to believe that these children will not be ragged at school with: 'Yah! Yah! Yah! You're only an IVF kid!' They may be persuaded that they are odd, in some way; and certainly, that mum and dad

[31] Gregory Pence, *Classic Cases in Medical Ethics*, 2nd ed., (New York: McGraw-Hill, 1995), p. 105.
[32] See Steptoe and Edwards, *A Matter of Life*.
[33] Gena Corea, *The Mother Machine*, pp. 150–53.
[34] Richard Blandau, '*In Vitro* Fertilisation and Embryo Transfer', *Fertility and Infertility*, 33 (1980), pp. 3–111.

were. Or conversely, they could become complete egoists, knowing that, in their generation, they stand apart from the rest of mankind.[35]

This seems to be an unusual argument, since it is essentially based on the publicity of being an IVF child. Such publicity would seem to only be a relevant consideration for someone like Louise Brown, the first IVF child, or possibly for the first IVF child in Australia, or the first IVF twins. It also seems unlikely, as is pointed out by Singer and Wells, that this publicity would be any greater than for any other famous baby, such as a member of the Royal family.[36] The fact that IVF children might be teased at school also seems to be a non-argument, given that most children at school are teased at some stage. Again, with hindsight, we can see that IVF children are not suffering the sorts of psychological problems that were originally suggested, and IVF has become part of the reproductive landscape.

Having discussed the objections that were presented to the use of IVF, it is now time to discuss the way in which these objections are modified by ectogenesis. The argument against ectogenesis combines both of the aspects that we have just discussed. It suggests that there is no way of telling if children produced by ectogenesis will turn out to be normal, without actually producing an ectogenetic child. This is seen as an unjustified risk, with a completely unknown (and unknowable) chance of success. As Singer and Wells point out, studies on animals are unlikely to be helpful here, for it is really not physical damage, but psychological damage that is likely to result from producing a baby through complete ectogenesis. Jeremy Rivkin raised the possibility of psychological damage to the foetus in condemning IVF, but his argument seems to be far more forceful against ectogenesis:

> What are the psychological implications of growing up as a specimen, sheltered not by a warm womb but by steel and glass, belonging to no one but the lab technician who joined together sperm and egg? In a world already populated with people with identity crises, what's the personal identity of a test-tube baby?[37]

The difference between ectogenesis and IVF does seem to be quite significant here. In IVF, the embryo is only outside the uterus, in a laboratory environment, for a few days, and at a stage where the central nervous system has not even begun to develop. Ectogenesis would see the foetus growing in an artificial environment for months, including the entire period of development of the brain and nervous system. Without knowledge of the exact effects of the maternal environment on the foetus, it would seem that it would be necessary to try to mimic the entire uterine experience. The success or failure of such attempts, and the possible negative effects on the psychology of the ectogenetic child could really only be assessed in a human being.

---

[35] Laurence Fitzgerald, 'Test Tube Morality in the Final Analysis', *The Advocate*, (Melbourne) 5 April, 1982.

[36] Peter Singer and Deane Wells, *The Reproduction Revolution*, (Oxford: Oxford University, 1984), p. 51.

[37] Jeremy Rivkin and Ted Howard, *Who Shall Play God?*, (New York: Dell, 1977), p. 115.

While purely physical development between humans and non-human animals is similar, there is really no comparison between the psychology of humans and any other species. IVF was used in farm animals, apparently without any increase in the rate of physical abnormalities, which suggested similar results would be likely in humans. However, these sorts of trials would not be able to evaluate the most important potential problem for the ectogenetic child, since it would clearly be impossible to assess the psychological damage that ectogenesis might cause to a sheep or a cow. It would seem that the only way to see if a child could develop normally after ectogenesis would be to produce human babies through ectogenesis, and see if they developed normally. This is especially problematic since although gross psychological problems might be immediately apparent, other less obvious problems, such as learning difficulties for example, might take years to manifest themselves.

This leaves ectogenetic research in something of a quandary, a problem that is noted by Singer and Wells:

> ... if it is unethical to attempt ectogenesis in humans until we have a reasonable assurance that it is safe, and we can have no reasonable assurance that it is safe until it is carried out, we seem to be in a classic 'catch 22' situation. Work on ectogenesis will remain forever unjustifiable.[38]

Singer and Wells suggest that the way out of this dilemma may be indirect research, intended to save the lives of premature newborns. As I indicated in the section on the scientific aspects of ectogenesis, I also believe that ectogenesis is most likely to be achieved through indirect research. If premature newborns are saved from earlier and earlier stages of gestation, then eventually the technique of ectogenesis may be discovered almost by default, without the necessity of any possibly unethical research on the unborn.

There is a third way in which it has been suggested that a child may be harmed by IVF. This is the fact that IVF and other reproductive technologies can be seen as unconsented-to experimentation on the unborn. This argument is a particularly potent one for the person who believes that all human beings, even embryos and foetuses, have a full right to life. This objection would seem to apply equally to IVF and to ectogenesis: if the experiments are unethical in the one case, then they will also be unethical in the other. However, if the embryo and foetus are not bearers of rights, then this objection is unfounded. If a being does not possess rights, then its consent to experimentation is unnecessary, for its rights cannot be violated. The question of whether embryos and foetuses actually do have rights is one that I will address in a later chapter.

---

[38] Singer and Wells, *The Reproduction Revolution*, p. 145.

Unnaturalness – The 'Playing God' Objection

Another objection to ectogenesis is that it is unnatural, sometimes phrased as 'playing God'. Singer and Wells have examined this objection, and distinguished a number of ways that ectogenesis might be termed 'unnatural'.[39] First, something may be unnatural if it is not what occurs in nature, untouched by humans. Second, something might be considered to be unnatural if it is not what occurs in the normal course of events. For example, people in the Middle Ages thought it was unnatural when people recovered from diseases that were usually fatal. This sort of unnaturalness was usually thought to be caused by magical powers obtained from the devil, and thus those who 'unnaturally' recovered from a usually fatal disease were often put to death. Third, something might be thought to be unnatural because it is not how God intended things to be. Fourth, something may be thought to be unnatural because it contravenes natural law theory.

Are any of these suggestions valid reasons to think that ectogenesis ought not be pursued? Let us examine each of them in turn. The first argument seems to be a complete non-starter, for two reasons: one, there seems to be no reason to exclude human actions from natural events; humans are mammals, so it would seem rather odd to suggest that the actions of dogs, cats, gorillas, whales, or chimpanzees are all 'natural' yet the actions of human beings are not; two, all human interventions are unnatural by this definition, which would mean that a person who rejects ectogenesis on this basis would be forced to also reject cars, computers, jet travel, medicine and telecommunications. While some things that humans do are certainly bad, there doesn't seem to be any reason to equate 'unnatural' with bad. In fact, there seems every reason not to equate the two terms, since doing so would mean that we would have to say that it was bad when a doctor saves a person's life through surgery.

The second definition of unnaturalness doesn't seem to be a good reason to reject ectogenesis either. Simply because something doesn't normally happen is no reason to think that it is bad when it does happen. The example that I used of the medieval people recovering from serious disease seems to be evidence enough that some things that are unnatural in this sense, are actually good things. Other examples might include spontaneous remission of cancer, a plane crashing and leaking fuel but not catching fire, and genuine free elections in a military dictatorship.

The third version of unnatural, and perhaps the most popular version of the argument, is that ectogenesis is unnatural because that is not how God intended things to be. This also seems to be a poor argument. It is open to two obvious replies. First, how can anyone know what God intended? Many people claim to have had direct revelation from God on many issues, but there doesn't ever seem to have been a consensus as to what God says on any issue. Usually the claimed revelation of one person will be in direct opposition to the claimed revelation of another. The second argument against this claim is that it is nothing more than appealing to the old suggestion that 'If God had wanted us to fly, He would have

---

[39] *Ibid.*, pp. 36–41.

given us wings'. This argument that ectogenesis is unnatural seems similar to the first argument that we considered. If ectogenesis is unnatural, then so is every other new development in human history.

However, there is a more sophisticated version of this particular objection that could be presented, based on the conservative view of abortion suggested by Dave Wendler.[40] His suggestion is that conservatives object to abortion because they see the process of foetal development itself as having moral significance, in that it is fundamental to the basic aspects of our lives, and they believe that it is important that this process proceeds essentially independently of human agency. If this is the view of abortion, then a similar view can be expected in regard to ectogenesis, since it could also be seen as an unjustified interference in the morally significant process of foetal development.

The problem with such an objection is that it assumes a vital premise in its argument: that the process of foetal development is morally significant. The objector needs to demonstrate this point, rather than to assume it. Unfortunately for the objector, the most likely defence of this position is the suggestion that this is not how God intended things to be, which leads us back into the less sophisticated forms of argument. Wendler's natural process argument may be an interesting new development for the conservative position (on both abortion and reproductive technology) but unless it is taken a great deal further, it will not really advance the position.

The last and most sophisticated argument for the unnaturalness of ectogenesis is that it contravenes natural law theory. Natural law theory suggests that over any laws that human beings may make to govern themselves, there is a coherent body of 'Laws of Nature' which can be ascertained (depending upon which particular version of natural law theory is being discussed) through intuition, the use of reason, or by study of the proper ends of natural things. According to this argument, ectogenesis is unnatural because it circumvents that natural order of things. This version of unnaturalness is also used to argue against contraception; contraception circumvents the natural order of reproduction by preventing conception, thus sexual intercourse is no longer serving its primary purpose, becoming instead merely a form of pleasurable activity. Pleasure is assumed to be a part of the function of the sexual orders, but not their primary function. The same objections that applied to the other arguments for the unnaturalness of ectogenesis can again be applied here, along with an additional objection: ectogenesis doesn't seem to be against the natural order of anything. Contraception circumvents the natural order of the reproductive system, but ectogenesis isn't part of that system at all. In fact, ectogenesis could be argued to be restoring the function of the system, in that it aims to overcome problems in reproduction.

Thus it would seem that none of the arguments against ectogenesis on the basis that it is unnatural give good reason to oppose the practice, unless one also wishes to oppose all other human innovations, including all other forms of medicine.

[40] Dave Wendler, 'Understanding the "Conservative" View on Abortion', *Bioethics*, 13 (1999), pp. 32–56.

Approaching 'Brave New World'

Another argument that has been proposed in opposition to the idea of ectogenesis, is that it will bring us one step closer to Aldous Huxley's dystopian vision of the future, that was presented in *Brave New World*.[41] This claim is undoubtedly true in one, trivial, sense – we don't currently have ectogenesis, the people of Brave New World do, and so creating ectogenesis would move us one step closer to the society portrayed in that novel. The more interesting and important question is whether this is actually a good argument for banning research into ectogenesis.

In order to assess this argument, some understanding of Huxley's vision of the future is necessary. Singer and Wells discuss this objection to new reproductive technologies, and they summarise the main aspects of Huxley's vision quite neatly:

> The family has been abolished. Every human being is conceived in a test-tube and gestation takes place in a laboratory. At nine months they are not born, but 'decanted'. Infancy and childhood are spent communally, and words like 'motherhood' are regarded as obscene. During childhood everyone receives intensive brainwashing, day and night. At night children receive 'hypnopaedic sleep teaching': an insinuating voice, throughout their sleeping periods, gives them moral instruction. They are taught that promiscuity is a moral duty, that the quest for pleasure is the purpose of life, and that the world they live in can hardly be improved. A rigid hierarchical structure is maintained by genetic engineering ... everyone ... is conditioned to be supremely happy with his or her station in life, and to wish for no other.[42]

The most important, and most fearful aspect of Huxley's vision, is the fiercely hierarchical structure, and the total lack of freedom. Huxley's futuristic society uses mainly negative interventions to ensure that everyone is happy with their place in the society. Many of the unborn foetuses are deliberately placed in hostile environments, in order to retard their development. This produces many people of lower intelligence, who are happy to perform the many menial tasks that are necessary for the smooth functioning of the society. It is only the fact that all reproduction is controlled by the state that allows this sort of intervention in the process of foetal development to take place.

Thus it would seem, as Singer and Wells point out,[43] that the most important way in which Huxley's future society is different from ours, is not the means of reproduction, but rather the power over every aspect of life wielded by the state. While ectogenesis might make it easier to manipulate the prenatal environment, the ability to do this will not necessarily lead us to *Brave New World*. Much more than ectogenesis is required to bring us to that point.

But surely there is more to it than this. The countries that lead the world in reproductive technology are countries with strong democratic traditions and laws founded on respect for individual rights. But not all countries in the world are like this. There have been, now and in recent human history, societies where virtually

---

[41] First published in Great Britain by Chatto and Windus, 1932.
[42] Singer and Wells, *The Reproduction Revolution*, pp. 41–2.
[43] *Ibid.*, pp. 43–4.

total control has been wielded by the government. If ectogenesis were to be developed, then the technology would spread through the world, and be available to any government that wished to use it. Another important point is that technology is not necessarily value neutral. Some technologies are designed for harmful purposes (napalm is probably a good example here). Other technologies affect the structure of the society that uses them: Singer and Wells point to the example of the microchip.[44] Development of a new technology like ectogenesis could have major effects on our society, and does have the potential to lead to a situation similar to *Brave New World*, if it is not used carefully.

Basically, this is a typical slippery slope argument, which suggests that the practices at the 'bottom' of the slope are so horrible, that we should not take even the first step onto the slope. A significant, but commonly unrecognised facet of such an argument is the fact that proponents of this type of argument do not have to concede the dubious point that the practices at the top of the slope are in themselves unacceptable. All that is necessary is to show that the allowing of such practices has the tendency to lead to other more unacceptable practices. Nor is it necessary for proponents of this type of argument to suggest that it is inevitable that we will slide to the bottom of the slope. If the practices at the bottom of the slope are reasonably likely to follow from practice at the top of the slope, and if the practices at the bottom are serious enough, then this would be enough to justify the banning of practices at the top of the slope. To give an analogous example, let us suppose that there is a ski slope that finishes with a very steep and dangerous section. Let us also suppose that we don't know how dangerous the rest of the ski slope is, but only that it ends with this dangerous section. Now if a choice had to be made between opening the slope to everyone or closing it to everyone, then I would suggest that the only responsible choice that could be made in those circumstances would be to close the slope to all.[45]

However, there are at least two other points that need to be considered here. The first point is that we are usually able to exercise some judgement about the slipperiness of the slope that we face. Not all slippery slopes are equally slippery. To return to the skiing analogy, we usually know quite a lot about the slope, apart from how it ends. If we can see that the whole slope is dangerous, then it is probably best to never set foot on the slope. However, if only the last section of the slope is dangerous, and one can easily stop before reaching that last section, then suggesting that no one should set foot on the slope seems somewhat over-cautious. The very fact that we are aware of the dangerousness of the end of the slope makes it that much more likely that we will avoid it.

The second point that needs to be made here is that not all slippery slopes are of even steepness, and there is often an obvious stopping point that prevents us from

---

[44] *Ibid.*, p. 44.
[45] The exposition of the slippery slope in this case is very similar to its use in other cases. Thus my description of slippery slope theory here is virtually identical to the description that I give in my 'Would You Like a Coffee? Slippery Slopes, Gratuities and Corruption in Police Work', *Professional Ethics*, 6 (1998), pp. 107–22.

reaching the dangerous section. Greg Pence pointed out this fact when discussing *Brave New World* in the context of whether IVF should be banned:

> The extension of Huxley's fictional ideas about psychological manipulation to 'genetic manipulation' and then to IVF – which is not genetic manipulation at all – was slipshod and misleading. Moreover, there was an ironic aspect to these citations of *Brave New World*, since Huxley had described the devastating consequences of loss of choice by individuals, and media arguments that IVF should be banned amounted to saying that couples should be denied a choice in this matter.[46]

Since it is the lack of respect for human autonomy that is the problem in *Brave New World*, it is this, rather than technologies like ectogenesis, that we need to be cautious of. The apparent slippery slope of reproductive technology seems to have a rather obvious stopping point: respect for personal choice and autonomy. As long as people are free to make their own choices about reproductive decisions, then the future of *Brave New World* will be avoided.

Feminist Discussions of Ectogenesis

The possibilities of the development of ectogenesis have been discussed by a number of feminist writers, most notably Shulamith Firestone, Julien S. Murphy, Leslie Cannold and Gena Corea. I wish in this section to give a brief overview of the main feminist positions and concerns about this issue, without providing an exhaustive listing of all the feminists writings on the topic. Many feminists have similar concerns about the development of ectogenesis, so discussion of a few writers is sufficient to highlight the most important issues.

The Feminist Case for Ectogenesis: Shulamith Firestone

The strongest supporter of the development of ectogenesis in feminist circles is Shulamith Firestone, who writes about the possibility in her book, *The Dialetic of Sex*.[47] In this work, Firestone argues that the root cause of inequality between the sexes is the natural reproductive difference between the sexes. The basic reproductive unit is formed of one male and one female, but the reproductive labour is not divided equally between them. Women must go through pregnancy and child birth, breast feeding and caring for the infants. This restricts their ability to be self-sufficient, and made them historically dependant on males for physical survival.[48] Firestone suggests that it is this unequal division of reproductive labour that has led to inequality between the sexes, rather than it being merely the result of upbringing and indoctrination as has been suggested by most feminists. While males can now take over the feeding and care of infants, pregnancy and child birth

---

[46] Pence, *Classic Cases*, p. 100.
[47] Shulamith Firestone, *The Dialectic of Sex*, (New York: Bantam, 1971).
[48] *Ibid.*, pp. 8–12.

are still the exclusive province of women. The solution to this inequality, suggests Firestone, is ectogenesis. This would allow the diffusion of the child bearing and child rearing role to the society as a whole, men as well as women.[49] The use of ectogenesis, according to Firestone, would allow women to be truly equal to men, since women would no longer be tied down by their own reproductive functioning.

Firestone also sees the end of pregnancy as a good thing in its own right. Even if women were truly equal with men in society without the need for ectogenesis, Firestone would seem to be committed to developing ectogenesis as a replacement for pregnancy. She describes pregnancy as 'barbaric', as 'a temporary deformation of the body of the individual for the sake of the species',[50] and as physically dangerous and painful. Moreover she describes birth in even less glowing terms, as 'like shitting a pumpkin'.[51] Relieving the pain and suffering borne by women in pregnancy and childbirth is an important ideal for Firestone, and ectogenesis could be justified merely in those terms.

In discussing Firestone's position, it needs to be recognised that she was writing in favour of a radical, new, equal society. Her revolutionary manifesto demands the removal of not only pregnancy and childbirth, but also capitalism, racism, sexism, the family in general, marriage, sexual repression, and all institutions that seek to keep women and children out of general society. The development of ectogenesis is merely a minor battle in this larger war of equality, and would achieve little by itself. Only in a society where all the other aims of this sexual revolution had been achieved could we expect the development of ectogenesis to be liberating for women. In isolation, all ectogenesis can do is to relieve some of the pain and suffering of pregnancy and birth: it would certainly not liberate women by itself. Firestone herself warns that 'in the hands of our current society, and under the direction of current scientists (few of whom are female) the attempted use of technology to 'free' anyone is suspect.'[52]

Firestone's arguments are used by Singer and Wells to support the idea that we should attempt to develop ectogenesis. However, the way that Singer and Wells use her arguments is actually inconsistent with the position that Firestone herself adopts. They advocate ectogenesis as a cure for infertility, but such a position is at odds with Firestone's rejection of the family and the importance of genetics. In Firestone's revolutionary society, ectogenesis would not be used to create descendants for the sake of any individual, but rather to create more children if (and only if) this was necessary for the good of society as a whole. The means of regulating the usage of ectogenesis would also be likely to come into conflict with Firestone's ideals. Since ectogenesis is likely to be a limited resource, it would probably exist on either (1) a 'user pays' basis which would make it available only to the rich, or (2) by government subsidy and available only to some persons, and even then only after careful screening. Neither of these alternatives would be palatable to Firestone. Since Firestone was seeking to remove all inequalities,

---

[49] *Ibid.*, pp. 233–4.
[50] *Ibid.*, p. 198–9.
[51] *Ibid.*
[52] *Ibid.*, p. 206.

including those of wealth, restricting ectogenesis to those who can afford it would obviously not be compatible with her ideals. Similarly, allowing access to ectogenesis only to those who passed certain screening tests, almost certainly based upon their ability to have children by other means, would be to privilege genetic parenting in a way that would also be opposed to Firestone's revolutionary ideas. Unless the entire basis of society was to change, ectogenesis would not be likely to be the attractive option for women that Firestone envisaged.

Firestone's ectogenetic solution can also be criticised on its own terms. Her solution to the inequality between men and women seems to be to eliminate all differences between men and women, in the hope that this will eliminate the reasons for the inequality. It does not seem obvious that the best way to deal with difference between men and women is to annihilate it. With this idea in mind, let us turn to other feminist criticisms of ectogenesis.

The Feminist Case Against Ectogenesis

Most feminists have written about the possibilities of ectogenesis in far less glowing terms than those used by Firestone. Some feminist writers have suggested that the development of some types of reproductive technology (including ectogenesis) might well be used as a means to get rid of women entirely. For example, Robyn Rowland writes:

> Much as we turn from consideration of a nuclear aftermath, we turn from seeing a future where children are neither borne or born or where women are forced to bear only sons and slaughter their foetal daughters. Chinese and Indian women are already trudging this path. The future of women as a group is at stake and we need to ensure that we have thoroughly considered all possibilities before endorsing technology which could mean the death of the female.[53]

This is certainly an extreme position, but it is not uncommon in some areas of feminist literature. Males are seen to 'put up' with females for the good of the species, but would prefer that they were not necessary.

Julien S. Murphy has pointed out that even if women were not necessary for reproductive labour *per se*, males would still wish to have them around for other reasons. She points out that nurture as well as pregnancy is primarily a female responsibility, involving not merely the specific task of child raising, but also nursing, elementary education, secretarial jobs and so on.[54] Females also tend to work more than males in necessary but tedious jobs such as electronic and textile manufacturing, and in cleaning and data processing.[55] She also suggests that male

---

[53] 'Motherhood, Patriarchal Power, Alienation and the Issue of 'Choice' in Sex Preselection', in Patricia Spallone and Deborah Lynn Steinberg (eds), *Made to Order: The Myth of Reproductive and Genetic Progress*, (Oxford: Pergamon, 1987), p. 75.
[54] 'Is Pregnancy Necessary? Feminist Concerns About Ectogenesis', in Helen Bequaert Holmes and Laura M. Purdy (eds), *Feminist Perspectives in Medical Ethics* (Bloomington: Indiana University, 1992), p. 190.
[55] *Ibid.*

egoism is maintained by the existence of females in a patriarchal culture, and that females are objects of sexual desire for many males, further reasons that suggest that even if it were possible to rid society of women, that this course of action would be unlikely to be followed.[56]

In fact, with our current technology and state of scientific knowledge, it would actually be easier to eliminate men than women. If ectogenesis was to be developed, and cloning by current methods was to be perfected for humans, there would still be a need for women in reproduction, but there would no longer be a need for men. What we currently call cloning, and what was actually done in the case of Dolly the sheep, is technically known as somatic cell nuclear transfer, or SCNT. In this process (in strictly non-technical terms), the nucleus of a fertilised egg is removed, and the nucleus of an adult cell is inserted in its place. Thus in simple terms, an egg is still required, though a sperm may not be (since the 'fertilised' egg could simply be an egg that has begun to develop through parthenogenesis). Thus even if ectogenesis were to be developed, thus relieving humanity of the need for a woman to carry the foetus, a woman, or at least her egg, would still be required to get that foetus in the first place.

Another concern expressed by feminists regards the motives of those who would seek to develop an artificial uterus. Some writers have been quite specific in questioning the motives of researchers working towards ectogenesis. For example, Gena Corea suggests that the real reason that men wish to develop ectogenesis is so that they can be sure that they are really getting 'their' child.[57] However, even ectogenesis might not solve this problem, unless fathers are able to perform all the steps themselves, from obtaining the sperm through to implanting a fertilised ovum into the ectogenetic device, since there is always the possibility of a medical mistake, or simple fraud.[58] Other often criticised motives for seeking to develop an artificial uterus include the desire to use it for eugenic purposes, and to use it to restrict women's reproductive choices (the latter of these will be discussed in more detail in the next chapter).[59]

Another likely consequence of the development of ectogenesis would be a change in the area of legal responsibility for the foetus. This is pointed out by Leslie Cannold in the introduction to her book *The Abortion Myth*:

> If babies are no longer fully gestated in the bodies of their mothers, then it no longer makes sense to claim – as feminists do – that abortion is solely a woman's right because it takes place solely in a woman's body. While women could still argue that their

[56] *Ibid.*
[57] See *The Mother Machine.*
[58] As an example of this, one IVF doctor in the United States was found to have used his own sperm to fertilise the eggs of his patients (without obtaining their consent). See Pence, *Classic Cases in Medical Ethic*, p. 116.
[59] Another possible motive is rather more psychological. This can be neatly summed up in the comment made by one of my listeners when I presented a section of this thesis at a conference in Hong Kong. One of the female conference participants dismissed the desire to develop an artificial uterus as 'womb envy', and claimed that it was simply another version of the male desire to have the biggest penis!

ownership of their bodies gave them the right to decide whether or not they would choose ectogenesis in the first place, once their foetus was in the artificial womb, any number of 'interested parties' – genetic fathers, doctors, grandmothers-to-be – could also claim 'rights' to it. One nightmare scenario ... is that a pregnant woman ... chooses to evacuate her foetus to an ectogenetic womb in preference to bringing the pregnancy to term. When the tiny foetus is born, the doctor ... concludes that it is severely damaged ... while the woman wants to shut down her foetus's ectogenetic life-support, her estranged husband (the genetic father) argues strenuously for keeping the foetus hooked up. Court proceedings follow ... [60]

While some people might see the change in legal status as an advantage of ectogenesis, Cannold suggests that this is not the case, since there is some evidence that the fathers most likely to get involved in disagreements about the future of their could-be children are the ones whose motives are the most questionable.[61] Studies in several countries examining 'father's rights' movements have found that the men involved in such groups were not interested in equal rights with the mothers of their children, but rather wished to assert the father's traditional right to control his family.[62] However, this objection does seem to miss the point. If rights are to be taken seriously, then you cannot deny someone their rights merely because you think they will exercise those rights poorly. Cannold's argument seems to be analogous to suggesting that slaves should not be given the right to freedom because if they had the right they might make poor decisions. If the development of ectogenesis would change the current situation with regards to legal and moral responsibility, then that is something that needs to be borne in mind when ectogenesis is actually developed. But you cannot argue that this change in legal responsibility is a reason for *not* developing ectogenesis, unless you have an independent reason for suggesting that the current situation is appropriate, beyond the mere biological fact that at the moment foetal development occurs exclusively within women's bodies.

Conclusions: Feminist Discussions

Julien Murphy seems to provide the best summation of, and answer to, the feminist positions. Her suggestion is that the best way to ensure that reproductive technologies in general, and ectogenesis in particular, are used to benefit women, is for women to be fully involved in the development and use of these technologies. If this is the case, then women can ensure that most of the feminist objections to the development of ectogenesis are avoided.

In fact, the only real objection that women could seem to have against the development of ectogenesis, would be if its development was in some way

---

[60] Leslie Cannold, *The Abortion Myth*, (St Leonards: Allen & Unwin, 1998), p. *xxii*.
[61] *Ibid.*, p. *xxiii*.
[62] See C. Smart and S. Sevenhuijsen (eds), *Child Custody and the Politics of Gender*, (London: Rouledge, 1989), pp. 158–89 and pp. 51–76. Quoted in Cannold, *The Abortion Myth*, pp. *xxiii–xxiv*.

injurious to the notion of female rights. The most likely area for this to occur is in abortion, and it is this question that I will consider at length in the next chapter.

Chapter 5

Abortion, Ectogenesis and the Foetus as Person

Now that we have examined some of the general implications of ectogenesis, it is time to turn to some specifics. The development of ectogenesis has been recognised to have important implications for some specific issues in the area of reproductive ethics. Probably the most important of these specific implications is the effect that the development of ectogenesis would have on discussions of the morality of abortion. If an ectogenetic device was to be developed that could be used to continue a pregnancy that had already begun in the uterus of a woman, then this could bring about drastic changes to the way that we think about abortion. An ectogenetic device that could be used to continue an existing pregnancy would make it possible to separate two currently inseparable aspects of the abortion procedure: the removal of the foetus from its mother's uterus, and the death of that foetus.

This possibility was discussed by Singer and Wells in *The Reproduction Revolution*, though not in any great depth.[1] They noted that the development of ectogenesis may well win the support of those who are opposed to abortion, for it would allow a woman to choose to have an abortion, in that the foetus could be removed from her body, without this resulting in the death of the foetus. The foetus would simply be removed from the woman's uterus and placed in an ectogenetic device until it was able to survive completely independently. This 'solution' to the abortion problem seems ideal in some ways, in that it allows the woman to exercise her right to bodily autonomy, by choosing to remove the foetus from her body, while at the same time respecting any right to life that the foetus may have, since the removal procedure need not result in its death. Indeed Singer and Wells suggest that the development of ectogenesis may well mean 'the end of abortion',[2] and allow 'pro-choice feminists and pro-foetus right-to-lifers ... (to) embrace in happy

---

[1] Peter Singer and Deane Wells, *The Reproduction Revolution: New Ways of Making Babies*, (Oxford: Oxford University, 1984), pp. 134–6.
[2] *Ibid.*, p. 134.

harmony'.[3] This argument in favour of the development of ectogenesis has been dubbed 'the abortion reconciliation argument' by David James.[4]

Some writers, such as Leslie Cannold,[5] are appalled at the suggestion that the development of ectogenesis would be welcomed by those in favour of abortion rights. In order to understand why some writers would be so opposed to the idea, and to understand why the idea of ectogenesis has come to be seen as a solution to the abortion 'problem', it will be necessary for us to detour for a moment, and examine some of the arguments that have been proposed regarding the morality of abortion. For it is only through an understanding of the arguments regarding abortion, and the way that some of these arguments have come to be a basis for abortion laws, that we can understand the real significance of ectogenesis in this debate.

Abortion

Discussion of the permissibility of abortion was generally confined to religious arguments before the early 1970s. Early discussions of the morality of abortion focussed on two main areas: the consequences of allowing or disallowing abortion, and the moral status of the foetus. Those who argued in favour of allowing a woman to choose to abort either argued that better consequences would flow from allowing abortion than from disallowing it, or they argued that the foetus had no moral status, or little moral status, and thus that seeking abortion was not immoral. Those who argued against abortion asserted that the consequences of allowing abortion were worse than not allowing it, or they argued that the foetus did have significant moral standing, and thus that abortion was wrong.

For example, let us consider for a moment the offering of Richard Stith, 'A Secular Case Against Abortion on Demand'.[6] Stith suggests that while the foetus cannot be proven to be a person, it also cannot be proven that it is not a person. Given that it becomes a legal person, with full rights, at the moment of birth, we should err on the side of caution and assume that the foetus is a person from conception.[7] In making such assertions, he is concentrating on the personhood or

---

[3] *Ibid.*, p. 135.

[4] David N. James, 'Ectogenesis: A Reply to Singer and Wells', *Bioethics*, 1 (1987), pp. 80–99, p. 82.

[5] See her works, *The Abortion Myth: Feminism, Morality and the Hard Choices Women Make*, (St Leonards: Allen & Unwin, 1998); 'Women, Ectogenesis and Ethical Theory', *Journal of Applied Philosophy*, 12 (1995), pp. 55–64; and *Women's Response to Ectogenesis, and the Relevance of Severance Abortion Theory*, (Masters Thesis: Monash University, 1992).

[6] In Garry Brodsky, John Troyer and David Vance (eds), *Contemporary Readings in Social and Political Ethics*, (Buffalo: Prometheus, 1984), pp. 189–94, original published in *Commonweal*, 12 November 1971.

[7] *Ibid.*, pp. 189–91.

non-personhood of the foetus. He then goes on to discuss the consequences of allowing abortion 'on demand', which he takes to mean 'abortion given to anyone on request, provided only that it be medically feasible'.[8] This effectively means abortion at any time in pregnancy, for any reason. In this case, he suggests that serious consequences would be likely to follow legalisation of abortion on demand, and thus that it should not be allowed. Abortion, he suggests, requires justification.[9] Thus his paper examines both the status of the foetus, and the possible consequences of liberalised abortion laws in concluding that, at the very least, abortion should be regulated.

Another example is Roger Wertheimer's 'Understanding the Abortion Argument'.[10] Wertheimer attempts to explain the various positions on the issue of abortion, focussing on the problem of whether abortion should be legal. The main issue that he discusses is the status of the foetus, which he suggests is a moral issue, rather than a factual one.[11] His eventual conclusion is that abortions may or may not be moral, but that laws prohibiting abortion are immoral, because such laws would be an unjustified assertion of the state's power over its citizens.[12]

Wertheimer and Stith reach essentially opposite conclusions, but they do so by discussing exactly the same points: the status of the foetus, and the consequences of laws on abortion. Such arguments saw the abortion debate become fiercely divided, with little room for compromise. Fuzzy arguments about the long-term consequences of allowing abortion (which were obviously difficult to predict) and the lack of a clear moral boundary during the development of the foetus, meant the debate became stalled with neither side having any real possibility of producing a knock-down argument to persuade the other. It was at this point in the debate that Judith Jarvis Thomson introduced her new, controversial, and innovative argument.[13]

Thomson's argument was an attempt to side-step the traditional problems in the abortion debate, by conceding (for the sake of argument) the opposition's main point. Those who opposed abortion almost inevitably insisted that the foetus was human (and by this they meant a person) from the moment of conception, and was thus a full bearer of rights. Thomson's argument granted that the foetus had a full right to life, but despite this, she still argued that a woman had a right to an abortion. She suggested that even if the foetus had a right to life, this did not mean that it had a right to everything necessary to sustain life.

Thomson proposed the analogy of a famous violinist, who requires the use of someone's kidneys to save his life. As it happens, you are the only person whose

[8] *Ibid.*, p. 189.
[9] *Ibid.*, p. 194.
[10] *Philosophy and Public Affairs*, 1 (1971), pp. 67–95.
[11] *Ibid.*, p. 78.
[12] *Ibid.*, p. 94.
[13] Judith Jarvis Thomson, 'A Defence of Abortion', *Philosophy and Public Affairs*, 1 (1971), pp. 47–66, reprinted in Richard Wasserstrom (ed.), *Today's Moral Problems*, (New York: Macmillan, 1975), pp. 104–20.

blood type matches the violinist, so only your kidneys can be used to save the violinist's life. The Society of Music Lovers has kidnapped you, and had the hospital connect you to his kidneys, and now you are in the position of being connected to the violinist and confined to bed for the next nine months until he recovers.[14] Thomson suggests that while it would be very nice for you to decide that you will remain connected to the violinist, he has no right to use your kidneys, and you can disconnect yourself from him, even if this will result in his death.

Now famous violinists, unlike foetuses, unquestionably have a right to life. So what Thomson claims to have shown is that at least in some cases the right to life does not mean a right to all that is necessary to sustain life, for the violinist does not have a right to use your kidneys. This neat argument, if it is really analogous to pregnancy and abortion, shows that a woman actually has a right to an abortion, where abortion is seen as the removal of the foetus from her uterus. This was a large step forward for the pro-abortion movement in many ways, for previous arguments had really only suggested that a woman should not be prevented from having an abortion, or that she did nothing wrong in having an abortion. Thus in passing laws that allowed abortion, society could be seen as giving permission to women to have abortions, or perhaps granting them that privilege. Thomson's argument went one step further, allowing a woman to demand an abortion as a right. But this step forward comes at a cost, for the right to an abortion is no longer the right to secure the death of the foetus, but rather the right to foetal removal. Thomson is quite explicit about this point.

I have argued that you are not morally required to spend nine months in bed, sustaining the life of the violinist; but to say this is by no means to say that if, when you unplug yourself, there is a miracle and he survives, you then have a right to turn round and slit his throat. You may detach yourself even if this costs him his life; you have no right to be guaranteed his death, by some other means, if unplugging yourself does not kill him.[15]

Thomson possibly had late abortions in mind when she made this point, for it was (and is) quite possible in late abortions for the foetus to be removed from the mother's uterus alive and viable. By Thomson's argument, the woman only has a right to demand the removal of the foetus from her uterus, and if it does survive this procedure, Thomson is quite clear in saying that it would be impermissible to kill it. This line has since been taken up by many other writers, most significant among them being Christine Overall[16] and, to some extent, Mary Anne Warren.[17]

---

[14] *Ibid.*, pp. 105–106.
[15] *Ibid.*, p. 119.
[16] See *Ethics and Human Reproduction: A Feminist Analysis*, (Boston: Allen & Unwin, 1987).
[17] See 'The Moral Significance of Birth', *Hypatia*, 4 (1989), pp. 46–65, reprinted with a postscript in Richard Wasserstrom (ed.), *Today's Moral Problems*, (New York: MacMillan, 1975), pp. 120–136. Page references in this discussion will refer to the reprinted version. See also *Moral Status: Obligations to Persons and Other Living Things*, (Oxford: Oxford University, 1997).

Arguments such as Thomson's, that state that a woman has a positive right to removal of the foetus from her uterus, have become the most important arguments in favour of abortion. There are several reasons for this. One reason that arguments such as this have become so important is because they focus on women, who are, after all, the ones who are pregnant. Discussions that focus solely on the personhood of the foetus can (and do) ignore women completely, for the location of the foetus is irrelevant to such an argument.

Another reason that such arguments became important is the fact that they make a positive claim, rather than a negative one: that a woman has a right to an abortion, rather than that she merely does no wrong in having one. Arguments that focus solely on the personhood of the foetus, even if they support abortion on demand, can only really say that a person does no wrong in killing the foetus. Thus they make a purely negative claim. But arguments such as Thomson's are quite different. These sorts of arguments are making a positive claim, that a woman has a right to an abortion, and thus that she can demand that the state protect her from those who seek to prevent her from exercising that right.

There is also the fact, noted by Leslie Cannold, that rights are the predominant moral currency in Western society, so making an abortion claim in terms of rights gives that claim a legitimacy that it would not otherwise enjoy.[18] In addition, making an abortion claim in terms of rights empowers women in a way that no other claim can, since this moves the issue from one where women can be seen as 'victims' who must be protected from backyard abortionists, to a position where women are asserting control over their lives.[19]

Arguments emphasising the woman's right to an abortion have also become important because most abortion lobby groups, both those in favour of abortion and opposing it, are based in the United States of America. United States Federal Law asserts that a woman does have a (somewhat limited) right to an abortion, founded in the legal right to privacy. This was the famous 1973 *Roe* v *Wade* ruling.

Roe v *Wade* discussed the regulation of abortion in trimesters, making different ruling about the legal status of abortion in each trimester. In the first trimester, *Roe* v *Wade* rules that the abortion decision 'must be left to the medical judgement of the pregnant woman's attending physician'.[20] In the second trimester, the State may regulate abortion in ways reasonably related to maternal health, for example by insisting that all second trimester abortions be performed in hospital. In the third trimester, the State may prohibit abortion except where necessary to save the life of the mother. As Pence points out, the ruling says that the State *may* prohibit abortion, but it certainly does not have to. Thus it is possible for a State to pass laws that allow abortion on demand prior to birth. Such laws would enshrine a woman's right to abortion at any point in pregnancy. But the minimum right for

---

[18] Cannold, *The Abortion Myth*, p. 13.
[19] Carol Smart, *Feminism and the Power of Law*, (London: Routledge, 1989), p. 153.
[20] Quoted in Gregory Pence, *Classic Cases in Medical Ethics*, 2nd ed., (New York: McGraw–Hill, 1995), p. 151.

women in the United States is the right to abortion in the first and second trimesters.

Given that the law in their own country enshrines the right to an abortion, it is not surprising that US abortion lobby groups focus on this right in their campaigns and rhetoric. However, since the abortion debate is a multi-national one, the lobby groups have tended to become multi-national as well, bringing US campaigns and rhetoric into other countries with different laws. This appears to have had the effect of misinforming many people about the law in their own country.[21] The pervasive influence of American media and culture only reinforces the misapprehension that women in other countries also have a legal right to demand abortion.

As a matter of fact, in many countries women do not have a right to an abortion. In Australia and the United Kingdom for example, the law allows doctors to perform abortions if they believe an abortion is necessary to safeguard the health of the mother, but abortion remains technically illegal. What this means, is that even when an abortion is deemed legally permissible, it is the judgement of the doctor that is important, and not the rights of women.[22] This fact was made quite clear in a discussion of abortion law in Australia, commissioned by the NHMRC.

The legal status of abortion places an obligation on doctors (and others) to play a gate-keeping role. The intention of the legislators and judge who established this role was precisely to ensure that the decision rested finally in the hands of the medical practitioner, rather than the woman.[23]

Yet many, even most, people in Australia seem to think that the law enshrines a woman's right to abortion on demand. This misapprehension serves to keep rights-based talk at the forefront of the abortion debate even where the abortion law is not based on rights, but rather is based on the bad consequences of banning abortion.

In fact, rights-based talk on abortion issues is so pervasive in the debate in Australia that it is common to hear anti-abortion groups invoking rights to support their positions (in this case the right to life of the foetus), even though this is really not relevant to the law in Australia. Abortion in Australia is only permissible to protect the health of the pregnant woman, and is basically dependent upon the idea of self-defence: that one can harm an innocent if that is necessary to protect oneself. Given that abortion law is grounded in this way, it should be obvious that the foetus is already being recognised, to some extent, as a rights-bearing individual, for if it was not, there would be no need to invoke the principle of self-defence. I will expand on this point with a few examples.

There are various living things that I may (painlessly) destroy without needing to provide any justification; bacteria for example, or mosquitoes, or weeds, or feral cats. Such living things are not the bearers of any legal rights. However, there are

[21] Cannold, *The Abortion Myth*, pp. 9–10.

[22] This is the case in both those Australian states where there are specific laws regarding abortion, and in those states where the law has been set by judicial precedent.

[23] National Health and Medical Research Council, 'Services for the Termination of Pregnancy in Australia: A Review', *Draft Consultation Document, Sept. 1995,* pp. 35–6. Quoted in Cannold, *The Abortion Myth*, p. 9.

some creatures that do possess legal rights of a sort. In New South Wales (and in other states), there are various animals and plants that are protected by law: it is an offence to harm them. However, this legal protection will not apply in all circumstances, for there are exceptions in certain cases which allow these animals and plants to be harmed or killed. Self-defence is one of these exceptions. So if, for example, I slipped while standing near the edge of a cliff, and in the process of trying to stop myself from falling, I uprooted a protected plant, I would be able to invoke the principle of self-defence to forestall any attempt to prosecute me for damaging a protected plant. Similarly, if my child (or any child for that matter) was being savaged by a dingo, I could kill the dingo to protect the child, even though the dingo is a protected animal. Again, I would invoke the principle of self-defence (which includes the defence of others) to forestall any attempt to prosecute me. On the other hand, if the child was being attacked by a feral cat, I could again kill the feral cat to protect the child, but I would not need to invoke the principle of self-defence to ward off the threat of prosecution, for feral cats are not protected by law. Self-defence is only required as a justification in cases where a holder of legal rights is being injured or killed in order to protect someone else. If the creature being harmed in protecting another person is not a bearer of legal rights, then it is not necessary to invoke the principle of self-defence to give legal justification to one's actions.

Since the principle of self-defence is being invoked in Australian law to justify abortion, then it must be the case that the foetus is, to some degree at least, a bearer of rights. Thus to protest that the rights of the foetus need to be recognised in law is effectively to protest in favour of an existing law.

In practical terms, what this overwhelming dominance of rights talk has meant, is that abortion becomes seen *only* as Thomson proposed: the removal of the foetus from the woman's uterus. The death of the foetus thus becomes an unnecessary, and in fact unwanted, part of obtaining an abortion. In light of this, ectogenesis, if it can be used to continue an established pregnancy, becomes highly desirable, for it would allow the foetus to be removed from the woman's body without ending its life.

The Ectogenetic Solution

It is exactly this argument that Singer and Wells provide as a justification for developing ectogenesis. They point out the fact that an ectogenetic device that could be used to continue an established pregnancy should be very attractive to those who champion foetal rights, since not only would ectogenesis allow abortion without entailing the death of the foetus, but it would also allow us to assist those who spontaneously abort, those who commence labour prematurely, and in cases of difficult multiple pregnancy. They also note that if a woman's right to an abortion is based on a right to control her body, then merely removing the foetus from her body will satisfy that right.

If the feminist argument for abortion takes its stand on the right of women to control their own bodies, feminists at least should not object (to ectogenesis).

Freedom to choose what is to happen to one's own body is one thing; freedom to insist on the death of a being that is capable of living outside one's body is another. At present these two are inextricably linked, and so the woman's freedom to choose conflicts head-on with the alleged right to life of the foetus. When ectogenesis becomes possible these two issues will break apart, and women will choose to terminate their pregnancies without thereby choosing the inevitable death of the foetus they are carrying. Pro-choice feminists and pro-foetus right-to-lifers can then embrace in happy harmony.[24]

Given the rights-based model of the abortion conflict, this conclusion of Singer and Wells is not only perfectly logical, it is also merely a step further on than had been previously suggested. Remember that Thomson herself had been quite explicit in separating the death of the foetus from the woman's right to bodily autonomy. If we assume that the foetus is a person, then the woman only has the right to remove it from her body; she does not have the right to kill it. While Thomson's comments about women having no right to secure the death of the foetus seem to be primarily directed at late term abortions, they apply equally well to ectogenesis. Other writers before Singer and Wells had also recognised the logic of the bodily autonomy argument as falling short of giving a woman the right to secure the death of the foetus.

Consider for example the classic paper of Mary Anne Warren, 'On the Moral and Legal Status of Abortion'.[25] Her discussion focuses primarily on the status of the foetus, concluding that it is not a person, and should not be granted the status of a person. However, she recognises that the foetus is a potential person, and that this potentiality grants it some value.[26] While she suggests that this value is insufficient to override the rights of the mother (who is a person, and thus possesses the full rights that the foetus lacks), she concedes that this potentiality cannot be ignored.

For our current purposes, the most interesting remarks that Warren makes are included in the postscript on infanticide.[27] Warren suggests that infanticide is not equivalent to murder, but it is not permissible, at least at this place and time, because there are many other people who would be willing to care for an infant if its parents are unwilling or unable to do so. This care might be in the form of adoption, or by paying for orphanages, or by some other means, but as long as such care exists, it would be wrong to destroy an infant simply because its parents do not want to care for it. Warren suggests that the significant difference between abortion and infanticide is that in the case of abortion the rights of the pregnant woman must be violated if the life of the foetus is to be preserved, and that this cannot be permitted to happen. However, she is quite clear about the limits of the rights of the mother after birth:

[24] Singer and Wells, *The Reproduction Revolution*, p. 135.
[25] See Wasserstrom (ed.), *Today's Moral Problems*.
[26] *Ibid.*, pp. 133–4.
[27] *Ibid.*, pp. 135–6.

The minute the infant is born ... its preservation no longer violates any of the mother's rights, even if she wants it destroyed, because she is free to put it up for adoption. Consequently, while the moment of birth does not mark any sharp discontinuity in the degree to which an infant possesses the right to life, it does mark the end of its mother's right to determine its fate. Indeed, if abortion could be performed without killing the foetus, she would never possess the right to have the foetus destroyed, for the same reasons that she has no right to have an infant destroyed.[28]

Such remarks clearly apply to ectogenesis. If it is possible to remove the foetus from the mother's body, and place it into an ectogenetic device to continue the pregnancy, then this would not violate the mother's rights, and Warren argues that this must be done, assuming that other people are willing to bear the cost, both emotionally and financially, of such care.[29]

Those opposed to abortion rights also seem to be logically committed to welcoming the advent of ectogenesis. The overwhelming majority of objections to abortion are based on the fact that abortion kills the foetus. However, if abortion was to become a severance procedure, a foetal evacuation from the mother's uterus to an ectogenetic machine, then the foetus' life is preserved. Those opposed to abortion rights on the grounds that abortion entails foetal death can hardly object to a procedure that seems to respect the pregnant woman's rights *and* preserve the life of the foetus. In discussing this, I will consider two papers that have been written in opposition to abortion rights: those of Don Marquis and Richard Stith.

Don Marquis' highly influential paper, 'Why Abortion is Immoral'[30] contends that abortion is morally problematic because it deprives the foetus of a valuable future, a future like ours. Leaving aside the problems of the argument (which I will discuss in a later chapter), the development of ectogenesis does seem to deal with Marquis' objections. The foetus is only deprived of a future like ours if it is killed. Evacuation to an ectogenetic device does not kill the foetus, thus it is not deprived of a valuable future, and this sort of abortion, by Marquis' own argument, is not immoral.

Similarly Stith's argument focuses primarily on the bad consequences of legalising abortion which, he says, many people regard as murder.[31] Obviously abortion can only be considered murder if the foetus is killed. Abortion as an evacuation procedure would circumvent most, if not all, of the bad consequences that Stith discusses.

Of course, not all writers on the issue of abortion will be satisfied with abortion as solely the transfer of the foetus to an ectogenetic device. Several influential papers argue for abortion on other grounds, usually the lack of personhood of the

---

[28] *Ibid.*, p. 136.
[29] In later publications, Warren has taken a major step back from this position. See especially *Moral Status*, pp. 214–5. However, her first paper is undoubtedly her most famous, and the discussions in the postscript on infanticide have had far more impact on thinking than have her later publications.
[30] *Journal of Philosophy*, 76 (1989), pp. 183–202.
[31] 'A Secular Case Against Abortion', p. 192.

foetus, and the arguments of these papers would not be affected by the development of ectogenesis. For example, Michael Tooley argues that since the foetus is not a person it has no rights, and thus may be destroyed.[32] Since the location of the foetus is irrelevant to such an argument, the development of ectogenesis would make no difference to the argument, since the foetus lacks the necessary features for personhood whether it is in its mother's uterus, or in an artificial uterus.[33] However, such arguments have declined significantly in importance since the rise of women's rights arguments, which is what makes ectogenesis seem to be such a desirable solution to the abortion problem. So for the moment I will not be considering such arguments, but will instead proceed on the same basis as Thomson in assuming, for the sake of argument, that the foetus is a person, and see what conclusions can be reached about the use of ectogenesis, if we grant such a premise.

Given the relative positions of those in favour of abortion, and those opposing, ectogenesis appears to be the perfect solution. It isn't even a compromise, for both sides of the argument get what they (apparently) want: the woman gets to have the foetus removed from her body, thus respecting her rights, and the foetus continues to live. Ectogenesis would seem to be a win-win situation.[34]

The Problem of Ectogenesis

Not all writers are enamoured with the idea of ectogenesis as a solution to the abortion problem. Leslie Cannold is one writer who has focussed on the problems that ectogenesis brings to the abortion debate. Her work is based on interviews conducted with 45 women, all residents of Melbourne, Victoria, in 1992. The fact that she was working with such a restricted sample does make it difficult to generalise from her work, but the opinions expressed are nonetheless of considerable interest.

Cannold raised several questions with the participants of her interviews in an attempt to draw out their views on the morality of abortion and ectogenesis. The most important question, for our discussion, was the following:

> Imagine that you are two months pregnant. You do not want to raise the child or are unable to do so and thus must decide between having an abortion or carrying the child to term and giving it up for adoption. As you are considering these options, a doctor approaches you and tells you that you have a third option. Thanks to technology, it is now possible for you to abort your foetus without killing it. Your foetus can be extracted from your body and transferred to an artificial womb where it will be grown until it is

---

[32] 'Abortion and Infanticide', *Philosophy and Public Affairs*, 2 (1972), pp. 37–65.

[33] Peter Singer has also presented a similar argument, though not in *The Reproduction Revolution*. See *Practical Ethics*, 2nd ed., (Cambridge: Cambridge University, 1993).

[34] This is assuming that the risks of ectogenesis would be equivalent to the risks of ordinary abortion – a point that I will discuss later.

able to live outside of that artificial womb (at around nine months), then it will be put up for adoption. The doctor informs you that this procedure carries no more medical risk or inconvenience to you than the traditional abortion method. Would you choose this third option?[35]

Cannold's hypothesis was that women would find the ectogenetic alternative an unsatisfactory response to the situation. This was borne out by the responses of the interviewees. What was perhaps the most surprising aspect of this study, was that ectogenesis was rejected by both those in favour of abortion rights, and those opposed to them. If 'pro-choice feminists and pro-foetus right-to-lifers … (would) embrace in happy harmony'[36] over the prospect of ectogenesis, it would appear from Cannold's studies that the harmony would be in rejecting it as a satisfactory solution to the problem of an unwanted pregnancy.

Cannold's works are filled with quotes from the women that she interviewed; in many places she simply allows these quotes to tell their own story. In discussing her work, and the conclusions that she draws, I too will be drawing heavily on the words of the women that Cannold interviewed, since the ideas and opinions that they express form the only really non-academic discussion of ectogenesis. However, in doing this I am somewhat limited, for I have no access to the original material, and so can only draw on the material that Cannold presents.[37]

In Cannold's discussion of women's attitudes to ectogenesis, she considers the opinions of pro-choice women and anti-choice women separately, and then makes a comparison between the two.[38] In examining her work, and her conclusions, I would like to proceed slightly differently, and examine the opinions of all the women she interviewed together. However, I will divide the discussion into two sections, as I think that the opinions expressed by the women reveal two major types of concerns about the use of ectogenesis; first, concerns about the technology of ectogenesis, and second, concerns about the ectogenetic abortion as an alternative to traditional foetal termination.

---

[35] 'Women, Ectogenesis and Ethical Theory', p. 58. Cannold notes that, in actual fact, any evacuation procedure is unlikely to be as safe as current abortion methods, but the question was phrased in this way to focus discussion onto particular issues.

[36] Singer and Wells, *The Reproduction Revolution*, p. 135.

[37] I did discuss with Leslie Cannold the possibility of having copies of the transcripts of the interviews that she conducted. She was receptive to the idea, but eventually (and quite properly) refused, since the women interviewed had not given permission for the material to be passed on to a third party.

[38] For example, Chapter Four of *The Abortion Myth*, entitled 'The Good Mother', is divided into sub–sections, several of which contrast the opinions of pro-choice women and anti-choice women. These include such sections as 'Pro-Choice Women and Adoption'; 'Anti-Choice Women and Adoption'; 'When the "Solution" is the Problem: Pro-Choice Women Reject Ectogenesis'; 'When the "Solution" doesn't Totally Solve the Problem: Anti-Choice Women and Ectogenesis', and so on.

Concerns with Ectogenetic Technology

Many of the women interviewed by Cannold expressed concerns about the technology of ectogenesis; whether its use is a good idea, whether it could be trusted to work properly, and who would be responsible for it. While some of these concerns might be dealt with by long-term use of ectogenetic technology without any evidence of harm to the child, other concerns may not be so easily allayed. Most of these objections are familiar, and I have already considered them in the section that discussed general objections to the technology of ectogenesis. However, it is interesting to see that these objections are ones that are being raised by ordinary people when the prospect of ectogenesis is raised, for this suggests that these are genuine concerns that would need to be dealt with if the technology of ectogenesis was to come into general usage.

Several women in discussing the possibility of ectogenesis alluded to its 'unnaturalness', or even explicitly mentioned the fact that this was a step towards Huxley's *Brave New World*. Annette's comment was typical:

> I have a real repulsion for the technology ... I believe that we're getting so far away from the physical act ... from our humanity so much, our whole physicality of childbirth and child rearing and everything ... we are just getting totally away from our bodies ... [having children] is a natural act ... it's just really instinctive.[39]

Nellie's comment was similar:

> I just think everything seems to be so unnatural nowadays. It just seems too strange to be doing all these things.[40]

And Grace:

> ... you should really be returning to nature as much as possible ... we're just getting further and further away from the core of our existence. The more we intervene with nature, and nothing's more natural than birth, the more our society becomes stuffed up.[41]

This is an objection that I have already discussed. In the section dealing with general objections to ectogenesis I noted that the fact that something is unnatural certainly does not mean that it is bad, for all human advances such as life-saving technology and labour-saving devices could be considered to be unnatural. The objections to the technology of ectogenesis that were raised by the women mentioned above seem to be most closely related to the unnaturalness argument

---

[39] From Cannold, *Women's Response to Ectogenesis*, p. 31. All names used are pseudonyms supplied by Cannold.
[40] *Ibid.*, p. 51.
[41] *Ibid.*

suggested by Dave Wendler.[42] He suggested that the process of foetal development itself has moral significance, in that it is fundamental to the basic aspects of our lives, and it is important that this process proceeds essentially independently of human agency. This certainly seems to be the position that is being advocated here, with the women making explicit mention of how natural birth is, and how we are getting away from the core of our existence. However, as I noted before, for this version of the unnaturalness argument to be accepted, the premise that foetal development is morally significant needs to be proven, rather than assumed. Yet it does seem to be an important fact that a number of women interviewed by Cannold raised this issue. This suggests that it is a serious issue in society, and if ectogenesis were to be developed, there would likely be opposition to its use in some quarters.

Another issue raised in the interviews was the possibility of the technology going wrong in some way. This reflects to some extent the earlier concerns about the unnaturalness of the technology, but it also focuses on the possibility of unethical experiments being performed on the unborn. Take Jacinta's suggestion that:

... nobody now thinks that a baby that's adopted – did they chop it up. If you go through a scientific process like this, I think that is a distinct possibility. They may experiment with it in some way. They may – not chop it up – they might inject it with AIDS, but we'll never know.[43]

Miranda had the same thought:

It's like putting your baby up to be a bit of a guinea pig, you know, to see.[44]

While these women explicitly mentioned the possibility that those in charge of the ectogenetic technology might engage in unethical experiments, there was also the fear expressed that the children produced by ectogenesis might be abnormal in some way. Grace commented that:

We're not too sure what sort of human being results from growing in a machine rather than a warm safe environment.[45]

Emily's concerns were similar:

A baby two months is nothing almost, you can hardly see it ... you think of putting that ... into a machine, with all sorts of little electrodes and what have you stuck to it to actually make it develop into a proper foetus with every limb to it, and you don't really

[42] Dave Wendler, 'Understanding the "Conservative" View on Abortion', *Bioethics*, 13 (1999), pp. 32–56.
[43] *Women's Response to Ectogenesis*, p. 30.
[44] *Ibid.*, p. 52.
[45] *Ibid.*

know. I mean even now when children are born at 23 weeks gestation there are too many risks.[46]

Carey also agreed:

> How do you guarantee that you bring to life a child that is whole, that is nourished and emotional and spiritual and mental and whatever, as a pregnancy within the womb requires, if you attach it to some technology?[47]

While long experimentation and testing might allay some of these fears, the view expressed by Jacinta was that nothing could convince her that the technology was really 100 per cent safe.

> It might be physically normal, I don't necessarily think it would be psychologically normal. And nothing you could say would convince me.[48]

These comments reflect the problem that it is virtually impossible to develop the technology without at some stage taking the risk of producing a severely physically, or more importantly developmentally, disabled baby. As I suggested earlier, the most likely way for this problem to be dealt with is for the technology to be developed by indirect means, but even indirect means will still have a significant risk attached.

A third type of objection alluded to by the women interviewed is the suggestion that those in control of the technology would not care about the foetuses in the ectogenetic machines, thus leading them to make inappropriate or uncaring decisions about their welfare. Janet suggested that:

> If you have the baby at nine months and hand it over to the family, OK you've got the added worry of whether the mother is doing the right thing to your so-called baby. If you [put it into an ectogenetic womb] I would worry about: were they looking after the foetus properly? What if they did something to it, and then it wasn't alright? Was it being looked after the way the foetus would be with me before I hand it over for adoption?[49]

Nellie also worried about whether the scientists in charge could be trusted:

> You're just putting the baby completely at the hands of science ... I mean, you can't trust science, anything could go wrong, just putting it at the mercy of the doctors or whoever.[50]

---

[46] *Ibid.*, p. 29.
[47] *Ibid.*
[48] *Ibid.*
[49] *Ibid.*, p. 30.
[50] *Ibid.*, p. 52.

Marybeth was concerned with the issue of possible abnormalities:

> ... what happens to those babies who, after two months, develop abnormalities ... does [someone] have a right to say ... that we should terminate it because no one would want that baby. Who would have [responsibility] for the baby?[51]

While such fears may seem irrational, it is true that technology does not always get used in the way that it was originally intended. As I have already discussed, the mere fact that reproductive technology has been developed in countries with a strong democratic tradition does not mean that the technology will be limited to these countries once it has been developed. It is an unfortunate fact that things cannot be uninvented. The development of ectogenetic technology would make it that much easier to interfere in the normal process of foetal development, a prospect which may be tempting for some. Nevertheless, this seems to be merely a caution to those in charge of the technology and its use, rather than a reason to ban its use altogether. There is also the fact that those who would be supervising the development of those foetuses that were placed in ectogenetic uteruses would have no direct connection to the foetuses, and thus may not feel as responsible for them should any problems occur. This question of responsibility is an issue to which I will return later.

There was also a concern among the women that it would be men in charge of the technology, and that this would tend to diminish the status of women in society. For example, Elisa seemed to be worried that the ectogenetic uterus would be used to get rid of women entirely:

> It's just like saying, well women have their role but we can do it better.[52]

Alison also worried that men were taking control of all of the areas of life that were traditionally the domain of women:

> There's this new thing that a man can strap over his shoulder, like a boob, you can put the formula in and he can actually nurse the child with this artificial tit hanging off one shoulder. I mean, we are a bee's dick away from giving them a womb.[53]

Carey agreed:

> A soon as you start looking at a third option, you're taking away a woman's power. Now men control most of the technology, that's a fact, but women have to date controlled the right to have or not to have a child.[54]

---

[51] *Ibid.*
[52] *Ibid.*, p. 31.
[53] *Ibid.*
[54] *Ibid.*, p. 34.

Such comments reflect common feminist concerns with reproductive technology, especially resistance to allowing men to control the one domain of human existence where women have previously been unique: the area of gestation. While there has certainly been a marked lack of respect for the autonomy of the women who have been involved as patients in the development of reproductive technology, I am unconvinced that this particular argument really carries any weight against the development of ectogenesis.

Adoption and Ectogenesis

None of the objections that have been mentioned so far are new; I have dealt with them all in previous sections of this discussion. However, there is one objection to the technology that was raised by the women who were interviewed that *is* new. Many of the women interviewed, both those in favour of abortion rights and those opposed to them, objected to the use of ectogenesis because it is too much like adoption, and they rejected adoption as an appropriate response to an unwanted pregnancy. The previous objections to ectogenesis came from those on both sides of the fence, with very similar views expressed by all the women. In this case, while the use of ectogenesis was rejected by virtually all of the women, the reasons for that rejection differed. Pro-choice women felt that ectogenesis was not a viable solution, and that only abortion was a realistic option for women who did not want (or were unable) to keep the developing child. Anti-choice women on the other hand, while agreeing that ectogenesis was not a solution, felt that the only appropriate response to unwanted pregnancy was to accept the role of motherhood.

Let us consider the comments of the pro-choice women first. Frances was of the opinion that ectogenesis would not provide a solution to the problem of an unwanted pregnancy because:

> I still wouldn't be able to separate myself from the child because I still would have conceived the child. It would still be out there somewhere, so it's just adoption before you have the child.[55]

Callie and Charity expressed similar opinions:

> I think there is still an emotional tie there, I think you've still created a life, and you're still responsible for that life.[56]

> I just think that whole concept of the baby ... being out there somewhere is really hard on the mother.[57]

---

[55] *Ibid.*, p. 28.
[56] *Ibid.*
[57] *Ibid.*

In the end, most of the pro-choice women felt that the decision that was made in the case of an unwanted pregnancy was one that had to be made on behalf of both the mother and the child. For example, Carmen stated that:

> When you are pregnant, the baby and you are a unit ... when you talk to a mother that's pregnant, you are talking to a person who is more than just a person you might ask in the street who is not pregnant ... So it's not a question of you and the baby. You are making a decision for both of you as a unit.[58]

Charity felt that:

> ... my decision to have an abortion would be the decision I made to care for the child that was within me. So to have the child outside somewhere else would be more cruel to me than just ending it because it's giving the child no help. It's still just saying 'well, it's not my problem' ... when you have an abortion you are making a decision about your own body and about that human's life.[59]

Women opposed to abortion also generally rejected ectogenesis as a solution to unwanted pregnancy, and suggested that it carried the same problems as adoption. Grace's view could have been equally expressed by a pro-choice woman:

> I don't think the woman gives up the total identity of the child, and it's always 'I wonder what's really happened to the child, perhaps I can go have a look'. So she's still in turmoil ...[60]

She added:

> I say there are always people who are ready for a cop out ... and this is an easy cop out ... it negates their responsibility. They've taken the child and they've put it in a machine where someone else can rear ... the child, and at the end of nine months it will be another human being ...[61]

The idea that ectogenesis would allow abortion to become something like a prenatal adoption is not new. In fact, severance abortion by ectogenesis has actually been described as foetal adoption by Robert Freitas, who advocated the use of foetal adoption as a means of solving the problem of the debate over abortion:

> Assuming these techniques are available, unwillingly pregnant women have an alternative to foeticide or unwanted childbirth. The reluctant prospective mother simply visits the local Foetal Adoption Centre, undergoes surgery for the removal of her viable foetus, signs legal documents, and exits a free woman. At the same time, the developing

[58] *Ibid.*, p. 32.
[59] *Ibid.*, p. 33.
[60] *Ibid.*, p. 50.
[61] *Ibid.*, p. 53.

embryo is preserved … The elegance of this scheme is evident in its ability to placate both proponents and opponents of abortion …[62]

This is of course the same solution later proposed by Singer and Wells, though they do not so obviously link the matter to adoption.

The obvious question to ask then, is why these women found the similarity between ectogenesis and adoption unacceptable? The reason is actually quite simple; almost all the women interviewed rejected adoption as an appropriate response to an unwanted pregnancy. This rejection came from women on both sides of the abortion debate, those for and opposed to abortion rights, and for a similar reason. Women on both sides of the debate felt that adoption, in most cases, was an abrogation of the woman's responsibility to the potential child that she was carrying. Essentially, though the thought was expressed in different ways, all the women thought that once a woman had given birth to a child, she was responsible for it, and had to look after it.

This conviction was most commonly expressed as a fear about the relinquishment process, with women on both sides of the debate citing the anguish of giving up the child as the reason why they would not choose adoption. For example, Lily said:

> I would have an abortion because I don't think I could emotionally detach myself. Knowing that I've had a kid, that it's out there somewhere. I'd also have that nagging feeling 'what's it doing now?'[63]

Callie believed that only abortion could separate you from the responsibility for the child you had borne:

> No matter what you thought, there's life here, and you are in some way responsible. I just find that you are responsible for putting another person on the planet … they would have to come back or they'd be wanting their medical history or anything like that. You are still responsible for them.[64]

A number of anti-choice women said that they would choose adoption over abortion, but admitted that what they were really saying was that they would choose to keep the child, and that adoption really wasn't an option. Sarah was an example:

> I wouldn't have an abortion. I'd carry that baby but I wouldn't be able to adopt. I'd find some way to keep that baby … I just know myself, I really couldn't give that baby up. I really couldn't.[65]

---

[62] Robert A. Freitas Jr, 'Foetal Adoption: A Technological Solution to the Problem of Abortion Ethics', *The Humanist*, May/June 1980, pp. 22–3.
[63] *Women's Response to Ectogenesis*, p. 24.
[64] *Ibid.*, p. 25.
[65] *Ibid.*, p. 48.

Martina's response was the same:

> I've had two children, and before I had them I would have said I wouldn't choose abortion because I don't believe in abortion, I think it's wrong, and I just would have said adoption straight out as being the other alternative. But … I couldn't adopt a child either, because you do grow to love it so much. I've had to make that choice, with my second child, because we really couldn't afford it, but I decided to keep my second child because we just couldn't part with it …
>
> Q: So really the choice is keep it or give it up for adoption, but it's really just keep it?
>
> Yeah, basically …[66]

Jacinta summed up the problem:

> … it's interesting that now that we have so-called legal and safe abortions, adoption has really gone out. And I don't think it's necessarily just fashion, I think it is the real choice that people choose, not to give a baby up for adoption because it's the hardest option.[67]

All the women that Cannold interviewed seemed to be of the opinion that a good mother would raise any children that she brought into the world, that adoption was a real choice in theory, but not a real choice in practice.[68] For the pro-choice women faced with an unplanned pregnancy, the choice was between abortion and motherhood. For the anti-choice women, the only responsible decision when faced with an unplanned pregnancy was to become a mother, and raise the child, despite the odds. As we have already said, these women also rejected ectogenesis as a solution to an unwanted pregnancy, for precisely the same reasons as they rejected adoption. In fact, most of the women felt that ectogenesis was worse than adoption, due to the perceived risks inherent in using the technology.[69]

The rejection of adoption by anti-choice women in particular is interesting, because adoption is the alternative usually proposed by those opposed to abortion, since it preserves the life of the foetus. None of the usual conservative arguments against abortion carry any weight against adoption, for they are all concerned with the fact that abortion kills the foetus. For example, Marquis' famous argument, that abortion deprives the foetus of a future like ours, does not rule out transferring the foetus to an ectogenetic device, since this will preserve the life of the foetus, ensuring that it will have a future like ours.[70] Other arguments that have been

---

[66] *Ibid.*, pp. 48–9.
[67] *Ibid.*, p. 24.
[68] *The Abortion Myth*, pp. 97–100.
[69] *Ibid.*, p. 106.
[70] 'Why Abortion is Immoral'.

presented specifically suggest that adoption is a preferable alternative to abortion.[71] Yet the women interviewed by Cannold still rejected it as a real life option. This suggests that there is more to the abortion debate than is usually admitted.

There is another piece of evidence that confirms the idea that there must be more to the abortion debate, from the conservative point of view, than merely respecting the foetus' right to life. This is the fact that most of the anti-choice women interviewed by Cannold were willing to allow abortion in cases where the pregnancy was a result of rape or incest.[72] Many conservatives are willing to allow abortion in these 'hard' cases, but their willingness to allow abortion in such cases is logically inconsistent, for the moral status of the foetus is the same no matter how it was conceived. The fact that many conservatives will allow abortion in such cases gives an additional reason to think that there is really more to the abortion debate than the mere question of the relative rights of foetus and woman.

If there is some further aspect of the abortion debate that is not usually considered, then it would seem to be extremely important to know what it is. From the interviews conducted by Cannold, it would appear that this unconsidered aspect is the issue of responsibility, for the general reason that the women rejected ectogenesis and adoption was that both options failed to take seriously the woman's responsibility for the foetus.

Responsibility and the Foetus

Several writers have discussed the issue of the woman's responsibility for the foetus, and what this might entail. Cannold discusses the issue in regard to the thoughts expressed by the women she interviewed, and Steven Ross has also discussed it.[73] But perhaps the most in-depth discussion of this issue is to be found in Catriona Mackenzie's 'Abortion and Embodiment',[74] so it is with her discussion that I will commence.

Mackenzie distinguishes several different types of responsibility that are important in discussions of abortion. First she discusses *causal responsibility* by which she means:

> responsibility for the direct causal consequences of one's actions in cases where those consequences can be said to be reasonably foreseeable and where a person's actions were freely chosen.[75]

---

[71] For example, see John Morreall, 'Of Marsupials and Men: A Thought Experiment on Abortion', *Dialogos*, 37 (1981), pp. 7–18.

[72] *Women's Response to Ectogenesis*, p. 45.

[73] 'Abortion and the Death of the Foetus', *Philosophy and Public Affairs*, 11 (1982), pp. 232–45.

[74] *Australasian Journal of Philosophy*, 70 (1992), pp. 136–55.

[75] *Ibid.*, p.138.

In defining causal responsibility in this way, Mackenzie differentiates between actions that are free and those that are unfree. Thus some women will be causally responsible for their pregnancies, and others will not. The obvious example of a woman who she does not consider to be causally responsible for her pregnancy is a woman who has been raped.

I would like to take a moment to expand on the idea of causal responsibility, as I think that it is an important notion which has not been examined in sufficient detail in the current literature on abortion. Mackenzie points out this fact, but does not really deal with the implications:

> ... it is significant that in this whole debate about responsibility there seem to be only two possible ways for women to get pregnant. Either they are raped, in which case they have no causal responsibility for the existence of the foetus ... Or else they are not raped, in which case they are held to be fully responsible, in both a causal and moral sense.[76]

Recognising that there may be different degrees of causal responsibility allows for more fine-grained distinctions about the morality of various actions than is possible if such differences are not recognised. I would suggest that a full spectrum of causal responsibility can be articulated. At one end stands the woman who has been raped, who has no causal responsibility for the existence of the foetus, and at the other stands the woman who has intentionally become pregnant and thus bears full causal responsibility. In between fall the myriad of other cases, such as the contraceptive failure, the drunken one-night stand, the woman diagnosed as infertile,[77] and the risk taker. I would suggest that many people would consider the circumstances of the pregnancy to be of importance in assessing the morality of an abortion. Thus the case of contraceptive failure would be seen differently from the female athlete who deliberately got pregnant and then aborted because the hormonal changes thus induced would enhance her performance.[78] I will return to this point later in the chapter.

The second aspect of responsibility that Mackenzie discusses is the notion of *moral responsibility*, by which she appears to mean responsibility for the future

---

[76] *Ibid.*, p.140.

[77] Many people do not realise that the medical definition of infertility is essentially probabilistic. A couple will be diagnosed as infertile after having not fallen pregnant after a year of regular unprotected sex. This certainly does not mean that the woman is unable to have children, or that she is incapable of falling pregnant; it merely means that the chances of her not falling pregnant after that time are, in probabilistic terms, low. Thus there is still a statistical possibility of a woman who has been diagnosed as infertile falling pregnant. Many couples who are considered infertile under this definition will eventually have children without medical assistance.

[78] The case of the female athlete was raised in one of Cannold's interviews, and was subsequently discussed with other interviewees. See 'Women's Response to Ectogenesis', pp. 21–2.

welfare of the foetus.[79] When the women interviewed by Cannold state that ectogenesis (and adoption) are an abrogation of the women's responsibility to the potential child, it is clearly this aspect of responsibility to which they are referring. Mackenzie suggests that the conservative position seems to equate causal responsibility with moral responsibility, and to construe moral responsibility as a responsibility to become a mother.[80] This definition of moral responsibility makes sense of the cases where conservatives will generally allow abortion. In cases of rape, for example, where the woman is clearly not causally responsible, she is not morally responsible either. If she is not morally responsible, then she does not have to commit to maternity, and abortion is permissible. Similarly in cases of incest, the woman is not causally responsible, or at least not fully responsible (since in such cases consent for intercourse is not deemed to have been autonomously given), and is thus not morally responsible, and again abortion is permitted.

I should note at this point that not all conservatives will allow abortion in cases of rape and incest (especially rape). Whether this is due to them holding a more consistent position on the moral status of the foetus, or whether they think that women are actually causally responsible for getting themselves raped is impossible to say in many cases. Hopefully it is the former. I should also note that while conservatives will *allow* abortion in cases of rape and incest, they certainly will not *suggest* it, and many would think it admirable if the woman proceeded with the pregnancy despite the way the foetus was conceived.

Mackenzie's suggestion that the conservative position seems to equate causal responsibility with responsibility to become a mother, seems to be confirmed by Cannold. The anti-choice women in her interviews were quite clear on this point, as evidenced by their views on ectogenesis as a solution to an unwanted pregnancy. As Cannold says:

> Most of the anti-choice women were incensed by the possibility that a woman who chose ectogenesis might feel that she hadn't done anything wrong because she hadn't had an abortion ... The goal of anti-choice women in supporting a movement which seeks to make abortion illegal is not the preservation of 'innocent' foetal life, but the conscription of all women who have conceived to motherhood.[81]

Whether moral responsibility *ought* to be construed in this way is another matter entirely.

Mackenzie distinguishes two different aspects of moral responsibility. They are *decision responsibility* and *parental responsibility*. Decision responsibility means assuming a moral responsibility to make a decision (or decisions) about the future

---

[79] Mackenzie does not explicitly define moral responsibility in her paper, though she does define two aspects of moral responsibility: decision responsibility, and parental responsibility. I will discuss these aspects of responsibility shortly.
[80] *Ibid.*, pp. 138–140.
[81] *The Abortion Myth*, pp. 109–10.

relationship with the being whose existence you are causally responsible for.[82] Mackenzie suggests that many factors need to be taken into account in such a decision. This will include such things as whether the woman is in a position to care for this being (both during gestation and after birth), how its existence will affect others with whom the woman has a close relationship (possibly the father or other children) and whether the woman will be able to provide for the could-be child's physical and emotional needs. A woman who decides to carry through with pregnancy will assume parental responsibility, which involves 'a commitment to bringing into existence a future child'[83] with all that entails.

The point that Mackenzie is making is that decision responsibility and parental responsibility are separable aspects of moral responsibility, and that a woman can therefore accept moral responsibility without accepting parental responsibility. She may decide that she is unable to accept parental responsibility, and thus decide that the most moral course of action is to abort, and end the life of her could-be child.

Another important aspect of Mackenzie's discussion is her highlighting of the asymmetry in the positions of men and women in regard to responsibility in pregnancy. While a man is obviously going to have to be causally responsible in pregnancy, it is possible for men to avoid decision responsibility, in a way that is not possible for women. If intercourse results in pregnancy, then the fact that the foetus will develop inside that woman's body makes causal responsibility obvious to her, and thus decision responsibility will be inescapable for her. Now, while it is possible for the woman to not realise that she is pregnant, unless she has a spontaneous miscarriage, at some point decision responsibility will be inevitably thrust upon her. On the other hand, a man may be ignorant of his causal responsibility, since he may not even know that the woman is pregnant. Or he can avoid decision responsibility by denying causal involvement; he can choose to avoid decision responsibility in a way that is quite impossible for the woman.[84]

From her discussion of the various aspects of responsibility, Mackenzie draws two important conclusions. First, she asserts that due to the asymmetry between the sexes in relation to all types of responsibility, it should be the woman who ultimately makes any decisions regarding the fate of the foetus. While the man involved may have some input into the decision, Mackenzie believes that due to the fact that prior to birth the decision will have much more effect on the woman than the man, any conflicts prior to that point should be resolved in favour of the woman.[85] Second, she suggests that the fact that a woman has chosen to terminate the life of the foetus that is growing inside her does not mean that the woman has

---

[82] 'Abortion and Embodiment', p. 140.

[83] *Ibid.*, p. 141.

[84] As the sex education teacher at my (all boys) secondary school so magically put it 'Some blokes seem to think that pregnancy isn't a concern for them, since they've already come and gone.'

[85] *Ibid.*, p. 142.

relinquished moral responsibility for that foetus. To make that suggestion, she asserts, is to conflate decision responsibility with parental responsibility.[86]

Mackenzie's analysis of responsibility in pregnancy is useful in explaining the attitudes to abortion and motherhood of the women interviewed by Cannold. As I have already said, the anti-choice women seem to believe that the only way to assume moral responsibility for the foetus is to accept the burden of parental responsibility. The pro-choice women, on the other hand, clearly felt that seeking an abortion as a solution to the problem of an unwanted pregnancy was not to abandon moral responsibility for the foetus, but rather to accept moral responsibility through decision responsibility, while still choosing not to take on parental responsibility.[87]

Abortion and the Indirect Death of the Foetus

Perhaps the most important point made in Mackenzie's discussion is the distinction between decision responsibility and parental responsibility: that accepting moral responsibility for one's actions, and for the life of a possible future child, does not necessarily mean that one must become a parent. If this is true, and I agree with Mackenzie's claim that it is true, then this means that there must be some alternative to one's becoming a parent that still involves accepting moral responsibility for the foetus, and the child that it may become. Since adoption has already been rejected as a possible alternative, and this would seemingly include pre-natal adoption by means of ectogenesis, then the only remaining alternative is abortion that includes the death of the foetus. It seems that it is this type of abortion that the pro-choice women are demanding, not merely that the foetus be removed from their bodies, but that its life be ended. Indeed from reading the statements made by pro-choice women about ectogenesis, it seems likely that given a choice between evacuating the foetus to an ectogenetic device, or carrying the foetus to term, that many of these women would choose to carry the foetus to term. As Cannold says 'Ectogenesis, like adoption, was seen as problematic for these women *precisely because it preserved the life of the foetus*'.[88]

There is a good deal of evidence, quite apart from the interviews of Cannold, that women who seek elective abortions actually are seeking the death of the foetus. Several discussions of abortion mention cases where the child has been born alive after an abortion, and either allowed to die, or where active steps have been taken to end its life.[89] If the object of abortion were merely to end the pregnancy, then this object has been achieved whether the foetus survives the

---

[86] *Ibid.*
[87] 'Women's Response to Ectogenesis', pp. 23–43.
[88] *Ibid.*, p. 82, emphasis in the original.
[89] See, for example, Raymond Herbenick, 'Remarks on Abortion, Abandonment and Adoption Opportunities', *Philosophy and Public Affairs*, 5 (1975), pp. 98–104, especially p. 101.

abortion or not. Taking steps, either by act or omission, to ensure its death if it has been born alive, shows quite clearly that the intent of the abortion is not merely to end the pregnancy, but to kill the foetus. Foetal death is also obviously the aim in cases of abortion due to foetal deformity. The only possible reasons for seeking abortion in such cases is to end the life of the foetus. To suggest that in such cases women might simply be seeking to sever themselves from the foetus is implausible in the extreme.

Thus the problem with severance abortion theories, such as that proposed by Thomson, is that they simply do not reflect the desires of the women who actually seek abortions. Her solution to the abortion debate, while perfectly logical, seems to be out of touch with what women actually want. At this point in time, when we cannot remove the foetus from its mother's uterus without killing it, women seem to get what they want from abortion by default. But the development of ectogenesis would drastically alter the situation, bringing with it the possibility that the foetus might well survive to become a child, precisely the outcome that women seeking abortion want to prevent. So the question arises anew, whether there are situations in which it is appropriate and ethical for a woman to demand the death of the foetus, while still granting the premise that the foetus has the rights of a person from the moment of conception. Given this premise, it would appear that the death of the foetus would have to be brought about by indirect means, for it seems implausible to suggest that one might be able to directly kill a being that has the rights of a person, if this is not necessary to protect the fundamental rights of another person.

David James raises one possible way in which women might still be able to ensure the death of the foetus. In discussing Singer and Wells' abortion reconciliation argument, James notes that there is likely to be a significant difference between abortion and what he terms foetal transplant: transfer of the foetus into an ectogenetic device.[90] James points out that most current abortions are performed by vacuum aspiration, which is a relatively minor procedure that does not require abdominal incision or general anaesthesia, but does not remove the foetus intact from the uterus. Foetal transplant, James suggests, is likely to be much more like a caesarean section, since it obviously requires the foetus to be removed intact from the mother's uterus. This is likely to require general anaesthesia and major surgery at the very minimum. James suggests that while women may not have the right to demand the death of the foetus, they should have the freedom to choose a less risky and invasive abortion over a more risky and invasive one.[91] Thus by refusing the more elaborate and risky procedure, women would ensure the death of the foetus by default.[92]

---

[90] 'Ectogenesis: A Reply to Singer and Wells', pp. 86–7.

[91] *Ibid.*, p. 87.

[92] A similar argument has been made by Joan C. Callahan. She argues in favour of the use of potassium chloride injection to produce second trimester abortion, despite the fact that this will absolutely guarantee foetal death, because this procedure appears to be the safest method of abortion. See 'Ensuring a Stillborn: The Ethics of Lethal Injection in Late

There are at least two problems with this argument. The first, pointed out by Deane Wells in his reply to James, is that ectogenesis has not yet been developed, and so we do not yet know what the procedure for removal of the foetus will be like.[93] It may be that the procedure is not as different from current vacuum aspiration methods as we expect. Until ectogenesis and foetal transplant are developed, we simply don't know how invasive the transfer procedure will be.

The second problem is the fact that there is no guarantee that women would be allowed to choose the method of abortion, even if foetal transplant was significantly more dangerous and invasive than vacuum aspiration. The rise of the 'foetal rights' movement has led to a spate of forced caesarean sections in the USA,[94] and there does not appear to be any reason to expect things to be significantly different elsewhere. If foetal transplant could save the live of the foetus, then it appears almost certain that this would become the required method of abortion in most jurisdictions. One legal method of forcing women to undergo foetal transplant rather than vacuum aspiration abortion has already been suggested. In 'Remarks on Abortion, Abandonment and Adoption Opportunities', Raymond Herbenick suggests that abortion be seen as a case of voluntary abandonment, which would thus allow state intervention under adoption law. Herbenick suggests that:

> ... voluntary consent to a medical abortion is sufficient for the state to intervene by regulatory laws to provide opportunities prior to an abortion for adoption by interested citizens, or for the state itself to place the child in custody in utero as a ward of the state.[95]

The foetus could be considered viable by virtue of the fact that it could be carried to term by an ectogenetic device, and thus the state (in the USA at least), under *Roe v Wade*, could assert its interest in preserving life. Thus the state could require the woman to undergo foetal transplant rather than permitting vacuum aspiration and the death of the foetus, even if this procedure was more risky for the pregnant woman than ordinary methods of abortion.

Even if there was no legal means available to ensure that women chose foetal transplant over vacuum aspiration, there are other means available to ensure that this is the choice made by most, if not all, women. If hospitals and abortion providers only offer foetal transplant, then that is the only means of abortion that women will be able to utilise, unless they wish to find a backyard abortionist who

---

Abortion' in Joan C. Callahan (ed.), *Reproduction, Ethics, and the Law: Feminist Perspective*, (Bloomington: Indiana University, 1995), pp. 266–83.
[93] 'Ectogenesis, Justice and Utility: A Reply to James', *Bioethics*, 4 (1987), pp. 372–9, especially pp. 377–8.
[94] 'At least 36 cases of forced medical treatment have been reported in the courts in twenty–six states,' Cynthia R. Daniels, *At Women's Expense: State Power and the Politics of Foetal Rights*, (Cambridge MA: Harvard University, 1993), p. 33.
[95] *Ibid.*, p. 102.

will perform another service. This idea may sound absurd, but there is evidence that suggests that abortions will be performed by whatever method is preferred by the doctor, not the method preferred by the patient. For example, Cannold cites the example of second-trimester abortions in Australia, where saline or prostaglandin injection abortion methods are used, rather than the less risky Dilation and breech Extraction (D and X), which has been medically proven to be in the best interests of the pregnant woman.[96] Apparently the main reason that doctors are still using instillation methods is because D and X is very taxing on the provider, despite being preferred by the patient. If abortions really are performed by whatever method is preferred by the doctor, then I see no reason why the doctor's moral preferences, as well as physical preferences, might not play a part in their decision.

Given all of these problems, it does appear that if women want to ensure that abortion involves the death of the foetus, they need to have a direct justification for it. Indirect justifications, such as those provided by Thomson and James, will not be sufficient to ensure that the death of the foetus remains a part of abortion after the development of ectogenesis. However, it seems extremely unlikely that we could find a direct justification for killing the foetus if it has the rights of a person, so I will examine that particular premise in detail. Rather than merely assuming the foetus has the rights of a person, I will examine the moral status of embryos and foetuses, and try to determine if these beings do in fact have such rights.

---

[96] *The Abortion Myth*, p. 52. Callahan suggests that KCl injection prior to D and X is even safer for women. See 'Ensuring a Stillborn', p. 275.

Chapter 6

The Status of the Embryo and Foetus

There are at least three positions that must be considered when examining the moral status of the embryo and foetus. First, that all human beings possess full rights from the moment of conception (the conservative view). Second, that persons, and only persons, possess rights and since neither the embryo nor the foetus is a person, neither possesses any rights, including the right to life (the liberal view). Third, that while the embryo and foetus are not persons, they deserve a level of respect, which is generally considered to increase as the foetus approaches viability(the moderate view). In order to reach some conclusions in this matter, I will examine each of these three positions in turn, to see which is the most reasonable. In order to simplify the discussion, I will use the term 'developing human' in this chapter to refer to the entity under discussion for all stages from fertilisation to birth, unless greater clarity as to which stage of development we are discussing is called for.[1] Despite the fact that it is not in general usage, I will use this term to add some clarity to the discussion, for it allows all stages in the development process to be uncontroversially grouped together. Whatever characteristics the fertilised egg, conceptus, blastocyst, pre-embryo, pre-implantation embryo, embryo or foetus have or do not have, they are all, at least, genetically human, and in the process of development.

The Status of Developing Humans: The Conservative View

The extreme conservative view is that the developing human is a full bearer of rights from the moment of conception. The basis of this opinion is the fact that there is no significant dividing line between the various stages of development of the developing human, and thus a line drawn at any point in the development of the developing human must be an arbitrary one.[2] We cannot, for example, say that there is any morally significant difference between a developing human of seven months gestation, and a developing human of seven weeks gestation, nor is there any morally significant difference between a developing human of seven months

---

[1] This term comes from John Morreall's 'Of Marsupials and Men: A Thought Experiment on Abortion' *Dialogos*, 37 (1981), pp. 7–18.
[2] The following discussion of the conservative position owes much to Rosalind Hursthouse, *Beginning Lives*, (Oxford: Basil Blackwell, 1987), pp. 31–47.

gestation, and a newborn baby seven hours old. Therefore, the conservative suggests, any distinction that we attempt to make must be made on morally non-significant grounds, and thus must be considered to be arbitrary, and morally suspect.

To illustrate this point, let us consider a number of points in the development of the developing human, where people attempt to draw a moral distinction. To begin with, let us consider the moment of birth. Can this be considered to be a morally significant moment in the life of the developing human? There are two obvious reasons for suggesting that the moment of birth might be morally significant. First, it is the moment where the mother no longer has a bodily connection to the child, and thus is no longer the only person who can possibly take responsibility for its care. From the moment of birth onwards, any capable person can take responsibility for the care of the child; it is no longer solely dependent upon its mother. Second, birth marks the moment where the developing human becomes visible, and thus is able to be perceived by people other than the mother.

However, the conservative would suggest that it is quite easy to see that neither of these two reasons for giving significance to birth is really a morally significant difference. Compare an unborn foetus of 38 weeks gestation with a newly born baby of 28 weeks gestation. By any measure, the foetus will be more advanced than the baby: it will be larger, stronger, more mentally developed. To suggest that the moment of birth marks a morally significant point in the development of a human being would appear to be giving privilege to location. It is to suggest that the mere fact that the less developed baby is outside a uterus while the more developed foetus is inside a uterus means that the baby is intrinsically more morally significant.[3] This seems to be an extraordinary suggestion, for to suggest in any other context that differing location provided for differences in *intrinsic* moral significance would be ludicrous (though differences in location may be morally significant in some situations).[4] The conservative would suggest that this reason cannot be used to suggest moral significance in the act of birth.

The second reason for attributing moral significance to the moment of birth, the suggestion that it is at birth that the baby becomes visible, also seems to be unable to carry any moral weight. First, new technologies now make it possible for virtually anyone to 'see' the developing human inside the uterus before birth.

[3] Mary Anne Warren is one writer who has suggested that the moment of birth has moral significance, but she does not suggest that the moment of birth changes the intrinsic moral status of the foetus/baby/child. It is extrinsic factors that make the moment of birth morally significant for Warren. See 'The Moral Significance of Birth', *Hypatia*, 4 (1989), pp. 46–65, reprinted with a postscript in Richard Wasserstrom (ed.), *Today's Moral Problems*, (New York: MacMillan, 1975), pp. 120–136. Page references in this discussion will refer to the reprinted version.

[4] Differences in location may be morally significant in some situations (see Warren, 'The Moral Significance of Birth' for example), but a mere difference in location does not make a difference to the intrinsic moral worth of an individual – it simply introduces another factor into the moral equation.

Ultrasound and related technologies give 'visibility' to the developing human long before birth. Second, to suggest that mere visibility marks moral significance is to privilege sight over the other senses. The unborn cannot be seen, but they can certainly be felt, and heard. To stress visibility as a mark of moral significance seems no better than stressing location. Thus the conservative would suggest that visibility is not morally significant, and that the second reason for seeing birth as a morally significant event fares no better than the first. Given that both of these reasons seem to be unable to be carry any moral weight, the conservative would suggest that birth is not a morally significant dividing line, and that the moral worth of the developing human must be considered to be the same as that of a new-born baby.

Given that the conservative position can find no reason to see birth as a morally significant event, let us turn our attention to the second point commonly cited as a morally significant moment: the point of viability. This is the point at which the developing human is able to survive outside the mother's body, albeit with technological assistance. Does this point mark a morally significant dividing line in the development of the human life? The fact that from this point on the developing human can survive without maternal assistance does seem to be significant, but once again there are significant objections to this view.

The most obvious objection is that this view seems to again place moral significance upon location: in this case not the location of the developing human, but rather the location of the mother. For since the time of viability is dependent upon the level of technological assistance that is available, a developing human that is considered to be viable in one location will not be considered to be viable in another. In fact, the developing human may be viable at one point in time, and then not be considered viable a week later, simply because the mother has moved.

Let me illustrate this point with an example. A woman is 25 weeks pregnant, and is visiting a doctor at the Monash Medical Centre in Melbourne. Since the Monash Medical Centre has one of the most advanced Neonatal Intensive Care Units in the world, the developing human inside her would be considered viable. Now suppose that the woman leaves Melbourne, and flies to Papua New Guinea. Once she arrives in Papua New Guinea, she walks up into the highlands, where she remains until the birth. Since sophisticated medical assistance is not available in the Papua New Guinea highlands, when she arrives in the highlands her developing human would *not* be considered viable, and in fact would not be considered viable for almost three months. In fact, if this woman was to continue to travel regularly between Papua New Guinea and a major centre in Australia, then her unborn developing human could reach the 'point' of viability several times, becoming viable whenever she was near sophisticated medical facilities, and not viable whenever she returned to the remote Papua New Guinea highlands.

Such an example shows the problem of using viability as a moral dividing line, since viability, even more than birth, privileges location. Such an objection is ample reason for the conservative to dismiss the suggestion that viability marks a morally significant point in the development of a human being.

What about the third point that has been suggested, the point of quickening, when the mother first feels the baby move inside her? Is this a morally significant moment? Again, it would seem that the answer would have to be no. While traditional Catholic theology saw the moment of quickening as the point where the developing human acquired a soul, there seems to be nothing at all significant about quickening once you possess some understanding of human development. Ultrasound clearly shows that the developing human moves inside the uterus long before it can be felt by its mother, and mere independent movement doesn't seem to be morally significant in any case. If mere movement is morally significant, then it would seem that we would need to ascribe moral significance to plants such as the Venus Fly Trap, which exhibits independent movement. This is a conclusion that few people would be comfortable with.

Given that none of the commonly suggested points in the development of the developing human seem to be truly morally significant, the conservative suggests that one must consider the developing human to have the same moral significance throughout its development, from conception through to birth and beyond. They thus suggest that since a new-born child is considered to be a full bearer of rights, then the embryo and foetus must be considered to be full rights-bearers as well, and to have a full right to life from the moment of conception.

A somewhat more sophisticated version of the conservative position has been suggested by Don Marquis.[5] His suggestion is not based on accounts of personhood, or on the difficulty of drawing a morally significant dividing line at any particular point in pregnancy, but rather on the suggestion that it is wrong to kill developing humans because to do so deprives them of a valuable future.

Marquis' argument against abortion generalises from the case of the wrongness of killing adult human beings. He suggests that we generally consider it wrong to kill adult human beings because to do so would be to deprive them of a valuable future.[6] However, since (most) foetuses would develop into adult human beings, it appears that most foetuses also have a valuable future, which gives a *prima facie* reason for thinking it is wrong to kill (most) normal foetuses. Since abortion, at this point in time, results in the death of the foetus, then abortion is immoral.

Criticisms of the Conservative View

There are several ways in which the conservative position on abortion is open to criticism. First, the logic of the argument itself can be criticised. Second, there is the fact that the conservative position seems to give special status to *human* life, rather than considering any specific characteristics that the particular life in question has. Third, there seem to be some difficulties in drawing distinctions between abortion and certain forms (or possibly even all forms) of contraception, a distinction that many, though certainly not all, conservatives wish to draw. Fourth, there are difficulties with the position when discussing extremely young embryos,

[5] 'Why Abortion is Immoral', *Journal of Philosophy*, 76 (1989), pp. 183–202.
[6] Marquis notes that the situations where we do not consider it wrong to kill an adult human being (apart from cases such as self defence) are cases where the adult does not have a valuable future – in justified cases of active euthanasia for example. *Ibid.*, p. 191.

in that these embryos consist of only a clump of undifferentiated cells, that may yet divide into identical twins. Fifth, there is the specific criticism of Marquis' argument on the grounds of personal identity. I will examine each of these criticisms in turn, to see how significant they are, and what response the conservative might give.

The basic logic of the conservative position is that there is on the one hand a being that certainly has full moral status (a child for example), and on the other hand a being that will, by means of a gradual process of development, become a being with full moral status (a developing human – zygote, embryo or foetus). If a morally significant property is held at one end of the spectrum, but not at the other, then there must be a non-arbitrary point in its development that marks the point of acquisition. But no such point can be found. Therefore, conservatives conclude that the being *always* has full moral status. Rosalind Hursthouse points out that there is a flaw in this argument, for an argument that is identical in formal structure, but contains different premises can lead to a false conclusion.[7] The example she uses is a green patch that is left in the sun, and slowly fades until it is blue. There is no particular point in the change that marks the transition from green to blue, but it is false to suggest that it was blue all along. Thus in a similar way, she suggests that simply because there is no specific point where the moral status of the developing human changes, this does not mean that it has possessed full moral status from conception. The only possible reply to this objection would be to point out that merely because the structure of the argument is invalid, this does not necessarily mean that the conclusion is false. While this is true, it is hardly a convincing rebuttal.

What about the charge that the conservative position gives special status to human life? That depends somewhat on which particular version of the conservative position is under consideration, but it would appear that most versions of the conservative argument *do* give special status to human life, as opposed to other species. Peter Singer expresses the problem with most conservative arguments quite neatly:

The central argument against abortion from which we started was:

First premise: It is wrong to kill an innocent human being.
Second premise: A human foetus is an innocent human being.
Conclusion: Therefore it is wrong to kill a human foetus.

... we have seen that 'human' is a term that straddles two distinct notions: being a member of the species *Homo Sapiens*, and being a person. Once the term is dissected in this way, the weakness of the conservative's first premise becomes apparent. If 'human' is taken as equivalent to 'person', the second premise of the argument, which asserts that the foetus is a human being, is clearly false; for one cannot plausibly argue that a foetus is either rational or self-conscious. If, on the other hand, 'human' is taken to mean no

[7] *Beginning Lives*, pp. 36–8.

more than 'member of the species *Homo Sapiens*', then the conservative defence of the
life of the foetus is based on a characteristic lacking moral significance and so the first
premise is false.[8]

Singer (among others) has argued at length that mere species membership should
not determine one's level of moral significance, and that our special treatment of
human beings at the expense of many other species on the planet cannot be
justified.[9] Species membership, in and of itself, is not morally significant. What is
morally significant are the features that an individual possesses. As I have already
suggested, capacity for autonomy would seem to confer on one a right to have that
autonomy respected. Thus if we were to find the necessary capacities for autonomy
in a member of some other species, then that being should be granted greater moral
significance than a being that does not possess those capacities, even if the second
being is a member of the species *Homo Sapiens*.

Developing humans of the types that we have been discussing clearly do not
possess the necessary features for autonomy, and thus don't seem to be candidates
for a right to autonomy, or any of the other rights that I have suggested can be
grounded in that individual's autonomy. In fact early developing humans seem to
lack all morally significant characteristics, including the ability to experience pain,
and thus do not seem to be candidates for any rights at all. This fact certainly
seems to suggest that most versions of the conservative position are guilty of
giving unwarranted special status to human life. The possibility that the foetus may
have special status due to its potential to develop morally relevant characteristics
will be considered later.

How might a conservative answer this criticism? It is a matter of fact that all
the persons we know of are human beings – we don't know of any non-human
persons. Some people have argued that some of the higher mammals might in fact
be persons,[10] but no definite conclusions about that can really be drawn at this
stage. Since all the persons that we know of are human beings, and almost all fully-
developed human beings are persons, it could be suggested that it is reasonable to
extend the rights of personhood to all members of the human species. However,
such a claim cannot simply be asserted, it would require an argument, presumably
based upon the good consequences of protecting all human beings by the
mechanism of full moral rights. Such an argument would be, of necessity, quite
lengthy, and I have seen no sign of it whatsoever in the philosophical literature.[11]

---

[8] Peter Singer, *Practical Ethics*, 2nd ed., (Cambridge: Cambridge University, 1993),
pp. 149–150.
[9] See, for example, his famous *Animal Liberation*, (London: Jonathon Cape, 1975).
[10] For example, see Singer, *Practical Ethics*, pp. 110–17.
[11] The closest that I have seen to an argument like this is found in Mary Anne Warren's
Moral Status: Obligations to Persons and Other Living Things, (New York: Oxford, 1997),
pp. 164–6. However, Warren only argues for the extension of full rights to those members of
the human species who have the capacities for sentience. She does not argue that all
members of the human species should be granted the rights of a person. Michael Davis

What of the third criticism of conservative theories, that they have difficulty drawing distinctions between abortion and certain forms of contraception? The Intra-Uterine Device (IUD) for example, seems to act by preventing the fertilised egg from implanting in the wall of the uterus, and the 'Morning-after' pill seems to act in the same way. Thus it would seem that both IUDs and 'Morning-after' pills are actually forms of abortion, since they prevent the further development of an existing member of the species *Homo Sapiens*. Serious conservatives should therefore be just as vehemently opposed to the use of IUDs and 'Morning-after' pills as they are to abortion.[12]

In fact, the problem is more serious that it appears, since the conservative argument for full rights for all human beings is often not phrased exactly as it was by Singer, 'It is wrong to kill an innocent human being'.[13] Instead it is often stated as 'It is always *prima facie* wrong to take a human life'.[14] This suggests rather more than the fact that a zygote should have the protection of rights, and in fact suggests that it is wrong to end the existence of any human tissues (including individual gametes) as they are both human and living.[15]

A more serious objection of this type can be levelled against Don Marquis' previously mentioned argument. Alastair Norcross has argued, through a series of thought experiments, that Marquis is wrong in denying that contraception as well as abortion deprives a being of a future-like-ours.[16] So let us consider his objection to Marquis' position. Marquis considers four possible candidates as a subject of harm in contraception: (1) some sperm or other, (2) some ovum or other, (3) a sperm and an ovum separately, and (4) a sperm and an ovum together. He dismisses (1) and (2) since assigning the harm to some sperm or ovum is utterly arbitrary, given that there is no reason to assign to harm to the male gamete rather than the female, and vice-versa. He also dismisses (3) because on this alternative, too many futures are lost: 'Contraception was supposed to be wrong because it deprived us of one future of value, not two'.[17] Finally, he suggests that in case (4) 'There are hundreds of millions of sperm, one released ovum, and millions of

presents a similar (but somewhat less complete) argument in his 'The Moral Status of Dogs, Forests, and Other Persons', *Social Theory*, 12 (1986), pp. 27–59. Rosalind Hursthouse discusses the way that we ought to treat alien persons, and suggests that if it was to be discovered that some members of an alien species were persons, then it would be right to treat all members of that species as persons. But this is essentially an argument about giving aliens the benefit of the doubt. It is not an argument that all human beings should have the rights of personhood. See *Beginning Lives*, pp. 103–107.

[12] In fact, some conservatives are also concerned about the use of such contraceptives, most notably a number of those involved with the Catholic church. However, most conservatives are much more concerned with abortion than with contraception of any type.

[13] *Practical Ethics*, p. 149.

[14] See Marquis, 'Why Abortion is Immoral', p. 185.

[15] *Ibid.*

[16] In 'Killing, Abortion, and Contraception: A Reply to Marquis', *Journal of Philosophy*, 87 (1990), pp. 268–77.

[17] Marquis, 'Why Abortion is Immoral', p. 201.

combinations of these. There is no actual combination at all'.[18] This leads him to dismiss contraception as depriving a being of a future-like-ours because 'there is no nonarbitrarily identifiable subject of the loss in the case of contraception'.[19] Norcross concentrates on case (4), so I shall do the same (though there are problems with cases (2) and (3) as well, which I will discuss shortly).

Norcross points out that even though there is no non-arbitrarily identifiable subject of loss, this does not mean that there is no subject of harm. In a series of thought experiments he demonstrates that in exactly analogous cases involving the killing of actual persons (that is adult human beings), the mere fact that there is no non-arbitrarily identifiable subject of loss does not make a difference in thinking that the killer has done something seriously wrong. In other words, the fact that it cannot be determined exactly who has been killed does not change the fact that the killer has deprived someone of a future-like-ours.[20]

It has been suggested by Walter Sinnott-Armstrong that Marquis could respond to this objection by insisting that only organisms can have a valuable future.[21] Since the sperm and ova before fertilisation are not the same organism as the one after fertilisation, they are not what is being denied a valuable future. This may help Marquis refute the particular objection that was proposed by Norcross, but it opens Marquis up (again) to the objection based on personal identity, which I will consider in a moment.

The fourth objection to the conservative position points out the problems in knowing exactly what will happen to a developing embryo. There are several issues that need to be considered in this context. In order to understand them, it is important to also understand the processes that occur in the first few weeks after conception. I will therefore discuss these events, and some complications that can occur along the way.[22]

Let us commence our discussion with the moment of conception, when the sperm first enters the ovum. The problem is that conception in fact is not a moment, but rather a process that takes about 24 hours to complete. First, two *pronuclei* are formed, one from the sperm and one from the ovum. These two pronuclei are then drawn together, and eventually combine in syngamy, when the chromosomes of the two gametes are finally combined. A few hours later, the zygote will divide for the first time, and this process of division will continue for the next few days. Even at this stage, when cell division has taken place, we are

---

[18] *Ibid.*

[19] *Ibid.*, p. 202.

[20] Norcross, 'Killing, Abortion, and Contraception', pp. 270–71.

[21] Walter Sinnott–Armstrong, 'You Can't Lose What You Ain't Never Had: A Reply to Marquis on Abortion', *Philosophical Studies*, 96 (1997), pp. 59–72, p. 60.

[22] The following discussion is drawn from Karen Dawson, 'Introduction: An Outline of Scientific Aspects of Human Embryo Research'; 'Fertilisation and Moral Status: A Scientific Perspective' and 'Segmentation and Moral Status: A Scientific Perspective' all in *Embryo Experimentation*, Singer et al. (eds), (Cambridge UK: Cambridge University, 1990).

dealing with a clump of undifferentiated cells, loosely bound together inside the *zona pellucida* (the outer membrane of the egg), rather than with a clearly developed 'life'. For example, it is not possible to tell which cells will eventually form the embryo proper, and which cells will form the placenta. When the pre-embryo has reached the eight cell stage, 'compaction' begins, when the cells start to adhere to each other, and some cells are pushed towards the middle of the clump. Later in development it is those cells which were pushed towards the middle that will form the membranes and the embryo proper, while the outer cells will form the *trophoblast*, which burrow into the lining of the uterus, and form the embryonic part of the placenta. The *trophoblast* forms about four to seven days after fertilisation, as the *zona pellucida* begins to degenerate. Implantation in the uterine wall is completed at about 14 days after conception. Shortly before the process of implantation is complete, the inner cells begin to differentiate into those cells that will form the embryo itself, and those cells which will form the embryonic membranes. At around 15 days after fertilisation, the primitive streak (which will become the backbone) appears, and individual organs begin to form from different groups of cells.

What I have just described is the normal process of embryonic development, but there are several complications that can occur. At any time up until the appearance of the primitive streak, monozygotic twinning is possible, where the embryo splits into two (or possibly more) identical groups of cells, that then continue their normal, but now separate development, into identical twins. Another possibility is that two or more pre-embryos that have resulted from one or more fertilisations fuse together to form a single embryo. This is known as forming a chimera. Though there have been few cases of chimera formation documented, this does not necessarily mean that the process is uncommon. It may simply mean that most chimeras develop normally, and never come to medical attention.

Another complication that must be considered is the possibility of conjoined twins. Conjoined twins (sometimes called Siamese twins) are identical twins who have remained joined rather than separating into two entities. The attachment between conjoined twins may be superficial (involving only skin), or it may be major (involving limbs, organs or even the brain). The rarest form of conjoined twins is known as foetus-in-foetu, unequal conjoined twins where one twin actually develops inside the other, usually in the chest or abdominal cavity.

Of most interest in this particular discussion is when each of these events can occur. Monozygotic twinning is believed to only occur up until the development of the primitive streak, at around 14 days after fertilisation. Chimera formation is not well understood, but appears to conform to the same time limits as twinning does, up to about 14 days. Conjoined twinning, however, can only take place after the appearance of the primitive streak, and can apparently take place much later than this, especially when in the form of foetus-in-foetu. For example, in one well studied case of foetus-in-foetu, the separation of the engulfed twin apparently occurred some four weeks after fertilisation.[23]

What implications do these various things have for the conservative position on the moral status of developing humans? First, it is often said that developing humans should have full rights from the moment of conception. This ignores the fact that conception is a process, and not a momentary event. There is also a significant problem for conservative arguments arising out of the possibility of twinning, and the formation of a chimera. This is because the identity of the adult and the zygote is often stressed by those arguing for the conservative position. Yet the possibility of twinning, and of forming a chimera, seem to preclude any talk of identity until after this possibility has passed. This would appear (from the case of foetus-in-foetu) to be at least four weeks after conception. After all, one can hardly say that this zygote will be identical with a later adult, when we do not know how many later adults we will be dealing with.

The possibility of monozygotic twinning also seems to be an objection to Marquis' view of why contraception is not wrong. As noted earlier, in his discussion of contraception, Marquis rejects as a candidate for loss (3) a sperm and an ovum separately, since on this alternative, too many futures are lost: 'Contraception was supposed to be wrong because it deprived us of one future of value, not two'.[24] Yet the possibility of monozygotic twinning means that two futures-like-ours could arise from a single zygote. Does this mean that it is permissible to kill one out of each pair of identical twins, since this will not reduce the number of futures-like-ours that we expected? Surely Marquis would have to say that monozygotic twinning means that two futures-like-ours would arise from a single zygote, and that it would be wrong to destroy either of them. Yet he rejects this same suggestion in his discussion of contraception. The possibility of forming a chimera also seems to cause problems for Marquis, for now instead of one future too many, we have one future too few. Norcross uses this fact to criticise Marquis argument for rejecting (3), since he points out that the fusion of the sperm and ovum to produce only one future is similar in all important respects to the single future produced when two zygotes merge to form a chimera.[25]

For the sake of completeness I should mention that there is another possible means of conception that produces an objection to Marquis' view that contraception is not wrong, in this case his rejection of (2) some ovum or other. This is the fact that in some rare cases *in vitro*, a phenomenon known as parthenogenesis has been observed to occur. This is the development of the ovum without fertilisation by a sperm. Since it occurs *in vitro*, it is reasonable to assume that it may also occur naturally. No births are known to have resulted from this process, but it does make it a logical possibility that an isolated ovum might

[23] Y. Yasuda et al., 'Foetus–in–Foetu: Report of a Case', *Teratolog*, 31 (1985), pp. 337–41.
[24] Marquis, 'Why Abortion is Immoral', p. 201.
[25] Norcross, 'Killing, Abortion, and Contraception', pp. 271–3.

possess a future-like-ours, which would make it a candidate for loss, contrary to Marquis' suggestion.

How might the conservative answer these numerous objections? Some conservatives note the problem of monozygotic twinning, and suggest that the end of the implantation stage is crucial for moral status, because at this stage there is no longer any possibility of twinning occurring.[26] However, this response seems to ignore the possibility of conjoined twins, unless the conservative maintains, against all logic, that conjoined twins are actually one individual and not two.

Marquis could of course respond to the objection to his argument by maintaining that it is the fact that at least one valuable future is lost that is important, and the actual number of valuable futures is irrelevant. This does, however, defeat his own argument which attempts to differentiate between abortion and contraception. Perhaps he might respond to that problem by insisting, as Sinnott-Armstrong suggests, that only organisms can have a valuable future. But as we shall see shortly, that suggestion also leads to further problems.

Parthenogenesis also seems to be a problem for Marquis' argument. He could perhaps respond that the event is so unlikely that it can be discounted, but this is likely to lead to further problems. For example, one might object that the probability of fertilisation after intercourse between a man with an extremely low sperm count and a woman who only irregularly ovulates is also extremely unlikely. If parthenogenesis can be discounted solely on the basis of probability, and thus is not seen as depriving anyone of a valuable future, then by the same token an abortion after the unlikely fertilization of an ovum from our irregularly ovulating woman by our low sperm count man could also be discounted. I am sure that this idea would not appeal to Marquis.

Let us now turn to the fifth criticism of the conservative position, which is specifically a criticism of Marquis' argument, that to destroy a foetus is to deprive it of a future-like-ours, and that this is *prima facie* wrong. The criticism of this argument is one based on the philosophical study of personal identity.[27] Marquis makes the following claim in his paper:

> The future of a standard foetus includes a set of experiences, projects, activities, and such which are identical with the futures of adult human beings and are identical with the futures of young children. Since the reason that is sufficient to explain why it is wrong to kill human beings after the time of birth is a reason that also applies to foetuses, it follows that abortion is *prima facie* seriously wrong.[28]

[26] Paul Ramsey, 'Reference Points in Deciding About Abortion' in J.T. Noonan (ed.), *The Morality of Abortion*, (Harvard University: Cambridge MA, 1970) noted in Dawson 'Segmentation and Moral Status', p. 54.

[27] The basis of this criticism comes from two sources. First, from Peter McInerney, 'Does a Foetus Already Have a Future–Like–Ours', *Journal of Philosophy*, 87 (1990), pp. 264–8. Second, from a paper by Tim Bayne, 'Abortion and the Immorality of Killing: How Far Back do I Go?', presented at the International Conference on Applied Ethics, Hong Kong, December, 1999.

[28] Marquis, 'Why Abortion is Immoral', p. 192.

It is central to Marquis' argument that adult human beings have (except in some rare cases) a valuable future, and that it is *prima facie* wrong to deprive them of that future. Since I am an adult human being, I have a valuable future, and it has been wrong to kill me since I acquired the property of having a valuable future. However, the question that must be asked is when did *I* acquire the property of having a valuable future? How far back does my personal identity extend? Can my personal identity be extended back to the time before my birth? Was *I* a foetus? Was *I* a zygote?

The answer to these questions will depend on the particular theory of personal identity that one chooses to defend. However, the general consensus in modern times is that some form of psychological continuity theory is the most appropriate theory of personal identity.[29] No theory of psychological continuity will extend back in time beyond the beginnings of consciousness: in other words, the person begins when consciousness begins. Now since consciousness is a property that is acquired during pregnancy, and is not possessed at conception, it would appear that not all foetuses possess a future-like-ours, since a being lacking the capacity for consciousness, on a psychological theory of personal identity at least, cannot be identical with any future person. This suggests a much more moderate conclusion than that proposed by Marquis, namely that it is only *prima facie* wrong to kill foetuses once they have become conscious.

One possible response to this objection, again suggested by Sinnott-Armstrong, is that Marquis can emphasise the fact that his argument avoids the concept of personhood, and merely point out that the foetus is the same organism as the body into which it will later develop (if not aborted) even if it is not the same person. Unfortunately, I don't think that Marquis would be willing to pay the cost of a response like this. For if we start to worry about the loss of futures of all organisms, then we are going to be worried about a lot more things than simply abortion. We would have to be concerned about the loss of future due to the killing of every animal, bird, lizard, insect, bacterium, virus, and so on. The whole point of Marquis' argument is that the foetus is deprived of a valuable future, and the future is valuable because of its future projects, activities, experiences and enjoyments.[30] These sorts of future experiences are valuable to *persons*, not to mere organisms. The future is valuable because it is the future of a person, and thus personal identity cannot be removed from the argument.

There is a somewhat more sophisticated reply that Marquis could make. Since a human embryo that develops normally will develop into a person, Marquis could argue that the fact that it is not yet a person is irrelevant. It will become a person, and thus possesses a future-like-ours, and it would be immoral to kill it.

---

[29] For example, see Derek Parfit, *Reasons and Persons*, (Oxford: Oxford University, 1984) pp. 199–350. I have myself defended this view. See my 'Thought Experiments and Personal Identity', *Philosophical Studies*, 98 (2000), pp. 53–69. McInerney also advocates such a view in 'Does a Foetus Already Have a Future–Like–Ours', pp. 265–8.
[30] Marquis, 'Why Abortion is Immoral', p. 189.

Unfortunately this reply will not work either, for if only persons have a future-like-ours, then the fact that something will develop into a person does not mean that *it* has a future-like-ours, but rather that it will *develop* a future-like-ours. The fact that this organism will develop a future-like-ours is not a valid reason for thinking that it would be immoral to kill it.

Before leaving the conservative position, there is one more argument that I must consider. This is the argument presented by Dave Wendler in the journal *Bioethics*.[31] Wendler's view is unusual in that he suggests that not only do non-conservatives misunderstand the conservative position, but that conservatives themselves do not properly articulate what their own position is! Given this position, perhaps the most surprising aspect of his argument is its plausibility: Wendler's argument that most conservatives do not really understand their own position is actually quite convincing.

Wendler suggests that the standard conservative position, rather than being based on the personhood of the developing human, as is usually suggested, is actually based on the natural development process of the foetus.[32] His suggestion is that, for the conservative, it is important that the process of foetal development proceeds essentially independently of human agency, and that this process itself has moral significance, that it is fundamental to the basic aspects of our lives:

> As supporters of CV (the conservative view on abortion) see things, we must accept the fundamental structure of our lives ... Put differently, the fundamental structure of our lives place moral boundaries that we may, ethically speaking, not alter to suit our own aims or desires ...[33]

When laid out more formally, the argument proceeds from the premise that deliberate interruption of a natural process which helps define the fundamental structure of our lives is seriously immoral, through the premise that foetal development is one of these natural processes and the premise that abortion interrupt this process, to the conclusion that abortion is seriously immoral.[34] Wendler uses this argument to examine several other aspects of the conservative view on abortion, and on other questions of life and death, and manages to argue quite convincingly that it is the process of foetal development that is really the important aspect of the conservative position.

---

[31] Dave Wendler, 'Understanding the "Conservative" View on Abortion', *Bioethics*, 13 (1999), pp. 32–56.

[32] In many ways this view is similar to the one presented by Ronald Dworkin in *Life's Dominion*, (London: HarperCollins, 1995). Dworkin suggests that the conservative view on abortion and euthanasia is based on a 'detached' objection (that life is sacred and ought to be respected) rather than a 'derivative' objection (derived from a particular view about foetal status). If one sees the natural development process of the foetus as 'sacred' in some way, then Dworkin's and Wendler's views become almost indistinguishable.

[33] *Ibid.*, p. 38.

[34] *Ibid.*, pp. 38–9.

Wendler points out that those who favour liberalised abortion laws may also grant moral significance to the process of foetal development. The important question is the level at which this moral significance is placed: type or token. The liberal would suggest that the moral significance of foetal development would depend upon the token: the facts of each particular case; how the woman fell pregnant, her family and social situation, her state of physical and emotional health, her financial situation and other such issues. The conservative, on the other hand, would place moral significance on the type: foetal development helps determine the basic structure of our lives.[35] This debate over the level at which moral significance should be placed is an obvious objection to this view of the conservative position.

Another objection to this view is the fact that all medical interventions are interruptions of natural processes, some of which, like death and dying for example, will clearly be morally significant, and fundamental to the basic aspects of our lives. If it is always unjustifiable to interfere with a morally significant and fundamental natural process, then all medical interventions in the process of dying, to note only one example, will be seriously immoral. This would mean that it would be seriously immoral to perform CPR on a person who has had a heart attack, to use a defibrillator on a person whose heart has stopped beating, to use a ventilator on a person who is close to death from respiratory insufficiency, and so on.

The only way to get around this particular problem seems to be to suggest that sometimes it *is* appropriate to deliberately interrupt a morally significant fundamental natural process. The problem then changes to determining when it is and is not appropriate to interrupt a morally significant fundamental natural process, which can really only be answered by reference to some other standard, such as a view on the moral status of the individual involved. Thus to answer the question of whether abortion is an unjustified interruption of morally significant fundamental natural process, there needs to be a prior belief on the moral status of the embryo and foetus, which is precisely the problem that is being discussed.

Whether or not Wendler's view helps to answer the question of the moral status of developing humans, it does have important implications. If Wendler is right about the importance of foetal development in the conservative view on abortion (and on the moral status of developing humans in general), then this will have important ramifications in other areas, as he himself notes:

> ... the natural process argument against abortion is seen as part of a more general argument that we should not attempt to alter the naturally defined fundamental structure of our lives. Abortion is one way of doing this, thus, advocates of the natural process argument oppose abortion. However, given that there are other ways of altering the fundamental structure of our lives, the natural process argument should be relevant to other debates in bioethics.[36]

---

[35] *Ibid.*, p. 39.
[36] *Ibid.*, p. 51.

Wendler himself uses the natural process argument to examine *in utero* genetic engineering[37] however, for my current purposes the question of the conservative position on ectogenesis will obviously be far more important. If Wendler is correct, then it could be expected that conservatives would oppose ectogenesis as an undue interference in the natural processes of foetal development. As we have seen from the statements of conservative women interviewed by Cannold, this is actually the case.

The Status of Developing Humans: The Liberal View

The liberal position agrees with the conservative position in one respect: both suggest that there is no morally significant point in pregnancy that marks a change in the moral status of the developing human. However, the liberal position suggests that since there is no point of change in status during pregnancy, the developing human has no rights at all. Some liberals extend the lack of rights beyond birth, concluding that infanticide may be permissible.[38] Others find some moral significance in birth, suggesting that the change in relationship (rather than location) that takes place with the event of birth brings about a change in the moral status of the developing human.[39] However, the change in moral status is based on consequentialist considerations rather than rights.

The basic premise in the liberal argument is that the developing human does not possess the necessary characteristics for personhood, since it lacks self-consciousness. A being that lacks self-consciousness, it is argued, does not possess a serious right to life, though it may possess some other rights, such as the right to not have unnecessary pain inflicted upon it. Even the right to not be inflicted with unnecessary pain would not apply to the foetus when it is non-sentient. Liberals argue that simply because the developing human is a member of the species *Homo Sapiens* is no reason to believe that the developing human has a right to life, for species membership, as already discussed, is not a morally relevant consideration.

What *is* morally significant is that a being possesses the attributes of personhood, most importantly self-consciousness. Since these attributes are certainly not present at birth, but rather are acquired at some later point, the developing human (and possibly even the newborn infant) cannot be said to be a person, and thus does not possess a right to life.

The examples that I gave for the implausibility of birth, viability and quickening as morally significant events, are just as important for the liberal as they are for the conservative. Indeed, every argument that I presented for the

---

[37] *Ibid.*, pp. 51–3.

[38] The two most prominent liberals advocating such a position are Michael Tooley (see 'Abortion and Infanticide', *Philosophy and Public Affairs*, 2 (1972), pp. 37–65) and Peter Singer (see *Practical Ethics*, 2nd ed., (Cambridge: Cambridge University, 1993)).

[39] See Warren, 'The Moral Significance of Birth'.

conservative position applies equally, but oppositely to the liberal position. Liberals agree with conservatives that the commonly cited events of pregnancy (conception, viability, quickening and birth) are not morally significant, with the possible exception of birth (to which I will return in a later chapter), and agree that the moral status of the developing human does not change over the course of pregnancy. However, instead of suggesting that this means that the developing human must be accorded full moral value (that is a full right to life) they suggest that this means that the developing human should be accorded no moral value, or at the most minimal moral value (no right to life).

Criticisms of the Liberal View

Like the conservative position, the liberal position is open to criticism. However, I believe that the criticisms that can be levelled at the liberal position are not quite as devastating as the ones that confront the conservative position. The claims of the liberal position do seem to be able to be defended to some extent, though probably not to the extent that proponents of the liberal position would hope. The biggest difficulty for the liberal view is the problem of infanticide. If one proposes a personhood view to justify abortion, including the claim that the foetus is not a person, and thus not deserving of moral rights, then this almost inevitably means that new-born infants will not qualify for personhood either. If new-born infants are not persons, then it would appear that they do not have the rights accorded to a person, and thus that there is nothing wrong with infanticide.

   This view is strongly counter-intuitive. Most people feel that there is a great deal wrong with infanticide, which may well lead to them rejecting the liberal position, or at least the liberal position based on the lack of personhood of the foetus.[40] In recognising this, proponents of personhood views have usually had to resort to providing special justifications as to why infanticide is wrong, usually based on the bad consequences that can be expected to flow from permitting infanticide.[41] The difficulties with this aspect of the personhood theory have been pointed out by several writers. Don Marquis for example, in discussing arguments in favour of abortion, notes that:

---

[40] If the reason that you are considering the moral status of the foetus is to attempt to justify abortion, then there are other strategies that can be pursued, rather than simply concentrating on the personhood (or lack of it) possessed by the foetus. One can, for example, concentrate on the rights of the mother. See, for example, Judith Jarvis Thomson's famous paper 'A Defence of Abortion', *Philosophy and Public Affairs*, 1 (1971), pp. 47–66. This is a topic that I will be discussing in a later chapter.

[41] Such justifications are often derided as being based on 'mere consequences'. It should be pointed out that those providing such defences are often consequentialists, and thus view consequences as the only morally significant aspect that needs to be considered. To deride their responses as 'mere consequences' is to completely miss the point.

All of the major well-known versions of the personhood strategy entail that infants are not by nature persons. Thus, philosophers defending such strategies either have to argue that, contrary to our moral intuitions, infanticide is morally permissible, or else they have to provide a special *ad hoc* justification of the wrongness of killing babies. In my view ... such *ad hoc* justifications of the wrongness of infanticide persuade only those who wish to be persuaded.[42]

While what Marquis says is intuitively plausible, I would suggest that there may well be some justification in suggesting that our moral intuitions are not as clear cut as he suggests. In fact infants are treated differently from adults, and this includes treatment of infants in life and death situations. The types of cases that I wish to consider here are cases involving severely disabled newborns. These cases have attracted a great deal of attention, in both the scholarly and popular literature, and reveal a great deal about our rather confused intuitions in the areas of killing and letting die, and the personhood of infants.

The most common intuition that people seem to feel when discussing moral issues, is what might be called the 'YUK!' intuition.[43] It is the intuition that many people rely on when they hear about some new moral problem, and it alerts them to the fact that their intuitions tell them that what someone is doing is wrong. ('I hear some scientist is trying to create a new species by fertilising human eggs with chimpanzee sperm'. 'YUK! That's wrong!') One particular problem with our intuitions, and the 'YUK!' intuition in particular, is that we are often unable to determine what particular aspect of a multi-faceted problem has aroused this intuition. I would suggest that this is the case when we examine the treatment of severely disabled newborns.

Peter Singer is one philosopher who has argued that under certain circumstances we should allow infanticide of severely disabled newborns. For many people with whom I have discussed this problem, the mere mention of this idea invokes the 'YUK!' reaction, and the conversation ends. However, there are (at least) two issues involved here. One, whether newborns should ever be deliberately killed by (say) lethal injection. Two, whether all severely disabled newborns should always receive the maximum possible treatment for their condition. I would suggest that it is the first issue, and not the second, that invokes the strong intuitive reaction from most people.

There are many cases that we could consider in this regard,[44] but I would like to focus on one specific case, that shows the issues fairly clearly. This is the 1983

---

[42] Don Marquis. 'Justifying the Rights of Pregnancy: The Interest View', *Criminal Justice Ethics*, 13 (1994), pp. 67–81, p. 69.

[43] I owe this term to Rev. Dr Doug Fullerton, a colleague from the Bioethics Committee of the Victorian Synod of the Uniting Church in Australia.

[44] For example, the details of a number of cases of non–treatment of severely disabled newborns are discussed by Gregory Pence in *Classic Cases in Medical Ethics*, 2nd ed., (New York: McGraw–Hill, 1995). See specifically Chapter 7: 'Letting Impaired Newborns Die'.

case of Baby Jane Doe.[45] Baby Jane Doe was born in October 1983 on Long Island, New York, with multiple birth defects. These included *spina bifida* (a serious defect of the spinal cord that often leads to other complications, most commonly serious and recurrent infections, and mental retardation), hydrocephalus (fluid on the brain), a damaged kidney, and microcephaly (small head, which implies a poorly formed, or possibly non-existent, brain). Aggressive treatment of these conditions would involve acting to try to minimise any mental retardation, including draining the excess fluid from the brain and operating to close the wound that exposes the spinal cord. Not offering aggressive treatment would probably lead to the baby's death within a relatively short time.

Baby Jane Doe's parents decided against surgery, allowing only palliative care – food, fluids and antibiotics. When the story broke, massive publicity surrounded the case. A suit was filed by a third party on Baby Jane Doe's behalf, seeking the treatment. The lower court hearing the case appointed an attorney to act on Baby Jane Doe's behalf; against the wishes of her parents he authorised the surgery. The parents appealed, and won, the guardian appealed to a higher court, the US Federal government became involved ... and eventually the courts ruled in favour of the parent's right to make 'medically reasonable' decisions on behalf of their child.

The interesting part about the case, as far as our current discussion goes, is that the public and media support in the case was firmly behind the parents and their decision to refuse treatment, even though the media reports made it clear that this would probably mean the death of Baby Jane Doe.[46] This suggests that in some cases, people's intuition is that it is appropriate to take action that will lead to the death of an innocent child. Other similar cases where public support was more divided involved infants that were less severely disabled, but it is interesting that even in those cases opinion was divided, rather than simply being united against the parents who wished their baby to die. Some of these cases involved babies whose only significant disability was Down's syndrome, which hardly qualifies as a severe impairment.

Even the strongest opponents of non-treatment of impaired newborns make some exceptions. Take, for example, the former Surgeon General of the United States, Dr C. Everett Koop, who implemented the famous 'Baby Doe squads' to protect impaired newborn from 'discriminatory non-treatment'.[47] He issued a regulation that directed that all infants were to be given treatment, regardless of disability, yet he agreed that there were some cases in which he would not give life-saving treatment. He specified (1) *anencephalic* infants (born with only a rudimentary brain), (2) infants who had suffered severe bleeding in the brain such that they would never be able to breath without a respirator, and would never be able to recognise another person, and (3) infants born without a digestive tract, as being among those infants who he would allow to die.[48]

---

[45] See Pence, *Classic Cases*, pp. 181–4.
[46] *Ibid.*, pp. 194–5.
[47] *Ibid.*, pp. 179–80.
[48] See Singer, *Practical Ethics*, p. 204.

My point in discussing such cases is to compare the way that people think about the non-treatment of such newborns with the way that they think about the treatment and non-treatment of adults. I would suggest that it is inconceivable that opinion might be divided about whether it was appropriate to treat an adult who as the result of an accident received brain injuries and minor disfigurement that would be equivalent to Down's syndrome. In such a case there would be no question – treatment should, must, be given. Even in the case of an adult who received injuries that placed them in an equivalent situation to Baby Jane Doe (serious but non-fatal brain damage, kidney problems, and inability to walk), I think that the response would be the same. Koop's example of the infant with severe brain damage as a result of bleeding is another interesting example, for this situation is extremely similar to what is termed persistent vegetative state (PVS). Adults in PVS are treated, sometimes for decades, at an annual cost that can be over $100, 000 USD per year. One patient was maintained in PVS for nearly 40 years.[49]

This seems to suggest that the previously mentioned 'YUK!' reaction is not to the idea of infanticide *per se*, but is rather to directly, as opposed to indirectly, bringing about the death of a baby. To killing, rather than letting die. Yet since writers like James Rachels have presented a strong case for the position that the difference between killing and letting die does not in itself make a moral difference,[50] it would seem that when people agree with non-treatment of severely impaired newborns, they are agreeing in effect, to infanticide. Cases like the Baby Jane Doe case also seem to suggest that people are willing to countenance this sort of treatment of infants in cases where they would not countenance it for adults. This certainly suggests that they do treat persons and non-persons differently.

However, an important point to note here is that the idea that it is appropriate to allow some newborns to die is a specific intuition, rather than a general one. If the liberal position is correct, then it would seem that it would be permissible to allow *all* newborns to die, if that is the wish of the parents. Yet this is not what our discussion would suggest. People only seem willing to allow severely disabled newborns to die, which suggests that there are definite limits to the way that human beings who are non-persons can be treated. I would suggest that the reason that people are willing to allow severely disabled newborns to die, but are not willing to allow normal newborns to die, is that the ability of the severely disabled newborns to become persons appears to be compromised. This suggests that the potential for personhood is in some ways morally significant, a position that I will attempt to defend in the next section.

---

[49] Pence, *Classic Cases*, pp 25–6.
[50] James Rachels, 'Active and Passive Euthanasia', in Rachels (ed.), *Moral Problems*, 3rd ed., (New York: Harper & Row, 1979).

The Status of Developing Humans: The Moderate View

The moderate position, like the conservative position, suggests that the developing human is worthy of moral consideration. However, moderates do not grant the developing human the same moral status as adult human beings. There are two main positions that I will be considering here: the idea that the developing humans potential to become a person grants it some moral status, and the view that there is a developmental milestone reached during pregnancy that changes the moral status of the foetus.

Proponents of the first moderate view point to the fact that the developing human is not yet a person, but does have the potential to become a person, and suggest that this grants some moral worth to the developing human, though not the same moral worth that would be given to a person. The people who stress the importance of foetal potential usually suggest that the moral considerability of the developing human changes during pregnancy, increasing as it develops.[51] However, there are some who suggest that the moral worth of the developing human does not change during pregnancy, and remains the same throughout, despite the changes that are occurring.[52] Effectively what this second view of potential as unchanging means, is that the potential to become a person gives the developing human the rights of a person. This makes this particular argument virtually indistinguishable from the conservative position, and so I will concentrate on the argument that potential grants some moral worth, but that this moral worth increases during pregnancy.[53]

An obvious advantage of this version of the moderate view is the fact that it does take into consideration the reality of the increasing developmental complexity of the developing human. To ignore the vast difference in developmental complexity between the single cell of the fertilised ovum, and a 40 week foetus does seem to be to ignore something important. By suggesting that the moral status of the developing human changes, increasing along with developmental complexity, or achieving some moral milestone during pregnancy, does seem to be a reasonable solution to this problem.

The second moderate position that I will be considering suggests that there is a developmental milestone that occurs during pregnancy that grants greater moral

---

[51] For example, this seems to be the position advocated by John Bigelow and Robert Pargetter in 'Morality, Potential Persons and Abortion', *American Philosophical Quarterly*, 25 (1988), pp. 173–81.

[52] See, for example, Jim Stone, 'Why Potentiality Matters', *Canadian Journal of Philosophy*, 17 (1987), pp. 815–30 and Michael J. Wreen, 'The Power of Potentiality', *Theoria*, 52 (1986), pp. 16–40.

[53] While I will not discuss the arguments that potentiality grants a full right to life, I will of course make use of the arguments in favour of the importance of potentiality that these writers have used.

status to the foetus.[54] A good example of this view is presented by Bonnie Steinbock in her book *Life Before Birth*. She derives her position on abortion from what she terms 'the interest view'.[55] Steinbock's view is based on the claim that morality involves taking into account the interests of others. In order to take others into account, it is necessary to define *who* must be taken into account. Steinbock suggests that since it is the interests of others that are important, then only other beings that actually have interests need to be considered. As consciousness is a prerequisite for the possession of interests, only those beings that are capable of consciousness (though not necessarily those who are presently conscious) are morally considerable. This would include other adults, who have interests in many things, and animals, which can suffer and thus have an interest in avoiding suffering. On the other hand, things such as plants, rocks and automobiles do not need to be considered, because such things do not have interests.

If we think of interests as stakes in things, and understand what we have a stake in as defined by our concerns, by what matters to us, then the connection between interests and the capacity for conscious awareness becomes clear. Without conscious awareness, beings cannot care about anything. Conscious awareness is a prerequisite to desires, preferences, hopes, aims and goals. Nothing matters to nonsentient, nonconscious beings. Whether they are preserved or destroyed, cherished or neglected, is of no concern to them. Therefore, when we care for things, or do what is necessary to keep them in mint condition, we are not acting out of concern for *them*.[56]

The interest view thus only ascribes intrinsic moral status to sentient beings, which makes it very similar to other well known 'developmental milestone' positions, such as the position advocated by L. W. Sumner.[57] Non-sentient beings may have instrumental value, or there may be strong consequentialist reasons for protecting them, but they do not have any intrinsic value, and thus they cannot be plausibly asserted to be the bearers of rights. Since there is good scientific evidence that foetuses are not sentient prior to about 20 or 24 weeks gestation,[58] this means that prior to this time they have no intrinsic moral value. When sentience develops, the foetus gains moral status. In other words, the moral status of the developing

[54] L. W. Sumner, 'A Third Way' in Susan Dwyer and Joel Feinberg (eds), *The Problem of Abortion*, 3rd ed., (Belmont CA: Wadsworth, 1997). Also to a lesser extent Mary Anne Warren, *Moral Status: Obligations to Persons and Other Living Things*, (New York: Oxford, 1997).
[55] Bonnie Steinbock, *Life Before Birth: The Moral and Legal Status of Embryos and Foetuses*, (New York: Oxford University, 1992), pp. 9–42. Don Marquis has suggested that rather than deriving her position on abortion from the interest view, she derives the interest view from her position on abortion. See 'Justifying the Rights of Pregnancy' pp. 67–81. I will return to this criticism later.
[56] Steinbock, *Life Before Birth*, p. 14. Emphasis in the original. Note that Steinbock uses a specific definition of 'interest', which does not fully correspond to the way that the term is used in every-day language.
[57] See 'A Third Way', in *The Problem of Abortion*, 3rd ed.
[58] *Ibid.*, pp. 49–50.

human changes during pregnancy, with the late foetus having moral value not possessed by the embryo and early foetus.

It is important to realise that Steinbock's interest view does not say anything at all about potential. Rather it examines only the *actual* characteristics of the foetus, its sentience or non-sentience, when determining moral status. Thus objections to the granting of moral status on the basis of potentiality do not affect her argument as it stands. However, if Steinbock does make surreptitious appeal to personhood in defending her position, as has been claimed,[59] then this apparent advantage of her position will disappear.

Criticisms of the Moderate View

Is it important that the developing human has the potential to develop into a person? Some writers have suggested that mere potential personhood is of no concern, and that the fact that the developing human will develop into a person has no relevance to its moral status before that time.[60] Others take a different view.[61] Thus it is necessary for me to examine the arguments about the importance of foetal potential.

Peter Singer points out that a potential X certainly does not have the same value as an X, or all the rights of an X, and uses this as the basis of his argument to dismiss the importance of potential with regard to the moral status of the developing human.

To pull out a sprouting acorn is not the same as cutting down a venerable oak. To drop a live chicken into a pot of boiling water would be much worse than doing the same to an egg. Prince Charles is a potential King of England, but he does not now have the rights of a king.[62]

While these examples are all quite true, this does not show that the proposition that the potential of the developing human grants it some moral status is false. While it is true that a potential person does not necessarily have all the rights of a person, this does not mean that a potential person has no moral value at all. A potential-X does seem to have more value than a mere non-X. Prince Charles is not the King of England, but neither is he an ordinary person. The fact that he is a potential King of England means that he has some rights (and responsibilities) that an ordinary person does not. For example, Prince Charles was eligible to represent the United Kingdom in the ceremony for handing back the territories of Hong Kong to China, where an ordinary citizen of the UK would not have been eligible,

---

[59] Marquis, 'Justifying the Rights of Pregnancy'.

[60] Peter Singer is one writer who rejects the value of potential in the foetus. See *Practical Ethics*, pp. 152–6.

[61] For example, Catriona Mackenzie in 'Abortion and Embodiment', *Australian Journal of Philosophy*, 70 (1992), pp. 136–55.

[62] *Practical Ethics*, p. 153.

and probably neither would another member of the royal family who was a more distant heir to the throne.[63]

It is also important to note that two of the three examples that Singer uses in stating his case are extremes in the development of the entity in question, which does tend to present something of a false dichotomy. The acorn is to the oak what the egg is to the chicken, and what the zygote is to the adult: but potentiality theses tend to pay more attention to the later stages of uterine development, such as the third trimester foetus. A third trimester foetus is rather more like a sapling than an acorn, and more like an egg about to hatch than a new laid egg. The moderate suggests that this difference is important.

A common criticism of potentiality theses is that they are unable to differentiate between the potential of (say) a developing embryo, and the potential of the individual gametes which will form the embryo.[64] Since most people who present an argument from potential do want to draw this distinction, this does appear to be a significant weakness in the argument. Also problematic is that fact that it may be difficult to draw distinctions between a developing human and merely possible future persons. If the children that I could produce have rights, most especially a right to life, then it would appear that by using contraception I am denying them their rights as potential persons. This would suggest that abortion and contraception are morally on a par, which is certainly counter-intuitive. There are two main strategies to deal with these problems. First, to draw a distinction between those potential persons who are actually developing their potential and those who are not, and second, to introduce some notion of probability of realisation of potential into the account.

One means of dealing with the objection to potentiality is to attempt to draw a distinction between the 'potential to *produce* persons' and the 'potential to *become* persons'.[65] This is the distinction between those potential persons who possess only a logical possibility of becoming persons, and those who are actually in the process of becoming persons. A separated sperm and ovum, when considered together, could be considered to be a potential person. But they have the potential to *produce* a person, rather than the potential to *become* a person, since the sperm and egg need to combine in order to fulfil their potential to produce a person, a process which destroys the identity of two entities (sperm and ovum), and thereby produces

[63] This example was suggested by Anthony Kwok–Wing Yeung in his paper 'Mere Potential Persons and Developing Potential Persons', presented at the International Conference on Applied Ethics, Hong Kong, December 1999.

[64] These problems are discussed extensively in Singer et al. (eds), *Embryo Experimentation*, (Melbourne: Cambridge University, 1990), most particularly in Peter Singer and Karen Dawson, 'IVF Technology and the Argument from Potential', pp. 76–89 and in Stephen Buckle, 'Arguing from Potential', pp. 90–108.

[65] I owe these terms to Stephen Buckle. See 'Arguing from Potential', pp. 93–101. This distinction is also alluded to by other writers, such as Jim Stone, who draws a distinction between strong and weak potential – basically the same distinction as I have mentioned. See 'Why Potentiality Matters', pp. 816–20.

one new entity. The embryo, on the other hand, has the potential to *become* a person, for the process of development only makes changes to this particular entity. As Stephen Buckle puts it, 'the process of actualising the potential *to become* preserves some form of individual identity'.[66] This is not the case with the potential *to produce.*

While we can easily *say* that there is a distinction between something that has the potential to produce a person and something that has the potential to become a person, does this distinction actually make any sense in practice? I would suggest that such a distinction can be defended. Consider, for example, the argument against the importance of potentiality presented by Mary Anne Warren in her classic paper 'On The Moral And Legal Status Of Abortion':[67]

> Suppose that our space explorer falls into the hands of an alien culture, whose scientists decide to create a few hundred thousand or more human beings, by breaking his body into its component cells, and using these to create fully developed human beings, with, of course, his genetic code ... I maintain that in such a situation he would have every right to escape if he could, and thus deprive all of these potential people of their potential lives ...[68]

Using this argument Warren suggests that the right to life of an actual person outweighs the right to life of potential people by literally millions to one. In fact, the argument could be made even stronger, for it would seem that the space explorer does not have a duty to assist the aliens in cloning him even if the process will not kill him, will not be painful, and will only take a few moments. This suggests that the right to life of potential people is pre-empted by the space explorer's right not to be inconvenienced, or perhaps by the right not to be cloned.[69] Now while our discussion at the moment concerns moral significance, and not rights, it should be obvious that if the rights of a potential person can be so easily pre-empted, that this must mean that the moral significance of a potential person must be very small indeed.

However, the problem with an example such as this is that it seems to be more comparable to contraception than to abortion. The space explorer prevents lives from coming into existence, but doesn't actually kill anyone. Let us call this case, space explorer$_1$. Now consider another similar case, which I will call space explorer$_2$. In this case, the space explorer has been captured, and the aliens have already removed some cells from his body, from which they have produced thousands of embryonic clones, which, if left to develop, would become persons.

---

[66] 'Arguing from Potential', p. 95. Buckle notes that the identity that is preserved is not personal identity, but rather numerical identity.

[67] See Wasserstrom (ed.), *Today's Moral Problems*, pp. 120–36.

[68] *Ibid.*, p. 134.

[69] This point comes from Anthony Kwok-Wing Yeung, 'Mere Potential Persons and Developing Potential Persons'.

Our intrepid space explorer sees the opportunity to escape, but in order to make good his escape, he would have to destroy all of these embryonic clones.

I would suggest that the intuitions generated by such an example are unlikely to be as clear as in space explorer$_1$. This does not necessarily mean that the space explorer would be doing the wrong thing in trying to escape in space explorer$_2$, even if this meant killing a large number of potential persons. My point is simply that it appears to be a much more serious thing when the case involves entities with the potential to *become* persons, rather than when it only involves entities with the potential to *produce* persons, as was the case in space explorer$_1$.

A comparison of the space explorer$_1$ case and the space explorer$_2$ case seems to suggest a significant moral difference between something that has the potential to *produce* a person, and something that has the potential to *become* a person. Yet there are ways that Warren might respond to this argument, and assert that the difference between the potential to *produce*, and the potential to *become*, is meaningless. For example, Warren might suggest that what is significant in the space explorer case$_2$ is not the fact that the explorer would have to kill beings with the potential to *become* persons, but rather that what is significant is the fact that the space explorer will kill living things in making an escape, something that is not necessary in the space explorer$_1$ case. This would suggest that it is not the potential to *become* a person that is significant, but rather a 'reverence for life' principle. However, I don't think that this defence can fully explain the change in intuitions between the two space explorer cases. If we change the space explorer$_2$ case so that in order to escape our explorer must kill a large number of ants (rather than the embryonic clones), I think that most people would see this as unproblematic. Yet ants, like embryonic clones, are living things, so there must be something more than a reverence for life driving our intuitions in the space explorer$_2$ case. This leaves the conclusion that there is a significant difference between the potential to *produce* and the potential to *become*.

What of the second way of distinguishing between the potential of an embryo and the potential of the gametes that combine to form that embryo? Can we draw a distinction by recourse to the probability of that potential being realised? This idea has been discussed by Peter Singer and Karen Dawson:

> A more promising attempt to distinguish the potential of the embryo from the potential of the egg and sperm in their culture medium is openly to acknowledge a link between potentiality and probability, by relating potential not to the bare possibility of the embryo, or whatever other entity we are considering, becoming a person, but rather to the probability of this happening. This has the inevitable result that potential ceases to be an all-or-nothing matter, and becomes a matter of degree. Traditional defenders of the right to life of the embryo have been reluctant to introduce degrees of potential into the debate, because once the notion is accepted, it seem undeniable that the early embryo is less of a potential person than the later embryo or foetus.[70]

---

[70] Singer and Dawson, 'IVF Technology and the Argument from Potential', p. 83.

The fact that introducing the probability of realising potential inevitably brings degrees of potentiality into the debate may concern the conservative who is arguing for a full right to life of the embryo, but it need not concern the moderate, who is not. In fact the moderate may welcome the introduction of degrees of potential, for this gives some stability to the idea of increasing moral status. As the probability of potential personhood increases, so does moral status.

On a view such as this, there are some crucial obstacles on the path to realisation of potential, and successful negotiation of each of these stages would seem to increase the moral status of the resulting developing human. For example, one obvious obstacle is fertilisation: without it there can be no realisation of potential.[71] Another obvious step is successful implantation in a uterus (of whatever sort). Again, without this necessary step, there will be no realisation of potential. An argument such as this would seem to be able to draw a distinction between the individual gametes and the resultant embryo, and between implanted and non-implanted embryos.

Singer and Dawson note one possible objection to this argument: the technique of micro-injection of sperm.[72] In this case, since the sperm and egg are selected in advance, there would seem to be little difference in potential before injection and after: even the genetic make-up of the resulting potential person will have been determined before fertilisation. I would suggest that there are two answers to this particular argument. First, the process of fertilisation still has to succeed, which is not a certainty, so there is some difference in potential before and after injection. Second, this seems to be an argument that raises the moral status of the gametes before injection, rather than reducing the status of the post-injection embryo. The fact that this particular egg and sperm have been selected for this process seems to make them special in a way that is not true of most other gametes, though it is true of some. For example, eggs that have been removed from a woman for the purpose of in vitro fertilisation seem to be special in a way that eggs removed from a corpse for the purposes of experimentation are not.

Having discussed some of the criticisms of the moderate view based on potential, let us turn our attention to the second type of moderate view, stressing the importance of the particular developmental milestone of sentience. I wish to examine in particular the criticism levelled at the interest view of Bonnie Steinbock by Don Marquis.

Marquis criticises Steinbock's position on two grounds. First, he suggests that there are actually several versions of the interest view, and that Steinbock does not select the one defensible version, but rather the one that yields the conclusions that she wants.[73] Perhaps not surprisingly, Marquis considers the most defensible version of the interest view to be the one that considers the future well being of all those creatures with interests, a view that sees the foetus as being a creature with a

---

[71] For the purposes of this discussion, I am willing to classify the beginning of parthenogenesis as a form of fertilisation.

[72] 'IVF Technology and the Argument from Potential', p. 87.

[73] 'Justifying the Rights of Pregnancy', pp. 71–2.

future-like-ours.[74] I would suggest that there are plausible reasons for preferring a different version of the interest view from the one suggested by Marquis, but to examine these reasons would take me too far from my present discussion.

The second criticism that Marquis levels at Steinbock is that the interest view only entails a right to an abortion before eight weeks gestation, and that Steinbock smuggles in a personhood strategy to bolster her abortion views.[75] The reason that he levels this charge is that the interest view suggests that sentient beings have moral considerability, and eight weeks gestation is the known lower limit for the possibility of sentience. I would suggest that Marquis is somewhat overstating the case here, and that the interest view seems to entail a right to abortion for any reason up until about 20 or 22 weeks gestation, since it appears to be extremely unlikely that sentience develops prior to this point. However, Marquis also points out a more significant problem, in that sentience grants some moral considerability, but does not necessarily grant full moral considerability. The problem here is that the interest view says more about who does *not* count in terms of morality, than it does about the relative weights of those who do count.

The interest view states that those who do not have interests do not count morally, thus allowing us to draw a line around those beings that are morally considerable, and those that are not. But if sentience is the *only* criterion for moral status, and all sentient beings have equal moral status, then this would to lead to a number of conclusions that Steinbock, among others, would not want to endorse. For example, this would lead to the conclusion that the life of a normal adult human being is of equal value to the life of a chicken, since both are sentient beings. Thus a person who had to choose between saving another person and saving a chicken from an approaching fire, would be doing nothing wrong in electing to save the chicken. The only ways to resolve this problem would seem to be to allow graduations in moral considerability, the path taken by L.W. Sumner,[76] or to adopt some sort of multi-criteria analysis of moral status that allows one to give greater worth to the lives of persons, which is the solution proposed by Mary Anne Warren.[77] It would seem to be this multi-criteria analysis that Steinbock is introducing, and that earns the criticism of Marquis.

In order for a multi-criteria analysis to actually work, it needs to be fairly specific about the relative values of the different criteria, and I think that this is the main problem with Steinbock's analysis. She suggests that it is reasonable to value the life of a person over a non-person, and a sentient potential person over a sentient lacking the potential for personhood.[78] Marquis points out the essential problem with this analysis: that assigning relative value to different beings does not assign them any absolute value:

[74] *Ibid.*
[75] *Ibid.*, pp. 74–7.
[76] In 'A Third Way', pp. 108–10.
[77] See *Moral Status*, especially Chapter 6.
[78] *Life Before Birth*, p. 68.

... even if Steinbock's assertions are true, they are compatible with giving persons a value of 100 on some scale of value, chickens a value of 1, and, following her argument, sentient potential persons, such as babies, a value of 2. Accordingly, her claim that babies have greater value than other sentient beings is quite compatible, not only with killing infants, but with having them for dinner on the days one does not have chicken.[79]

This particular problem for the interest view does seem to be difficult to resolve, unless one arbitrarily assigns some absolute values. The potential view does not seem to have the same problem however, since the graduation from minimal moral status to full moral status corresponds neatly to the level of potential that has been realised.

The Status of Developing Humans: Conclusions

Now that we have examined each of the major positions on the status of developing humans in some detail, it is time for me to try to draw some conclusions. The lengthy discussion of the conservative position highlighted what I believe are insurmountable problems with the proposition that all developing humans have full moral status from the moment of conception, or even from some later point in pregnancy. The discussion of the liberal position, especially in regard to infanticide, leads me to believe that newborn infants and late gestation foetuses do have significant moral status, but that this moral status is not absolute: thus even newborn infants do not have the full moral status granted to persons. Thus it would seem that one of the moderate positions will be the most defensible. Marquis' objections to the interest view do seem to be substantial, thus suggesting that the interest view requires support from a personhood strategy, but Marquis fails to convince me that the personhood strategy is untenable. This then leaves the moderate position based upon the potential for personhood of the foetus. But what of the problems that have been suggested for the potentiality view? In order to deal with those, we will need to briefly re-examine some of the objections to the importance of potential.

Let us begin by returning to a previous example, the acorn to oak case suggested by Peter Singer. I suggested that a third trimester foetus is rather more like a sapling than an acorn, and that the change from a fertilised ovum to a third trimester foetus is significant. The acorn to oak analogy can probably be stretched to illustrate this point. Imagine that you want an oak tree in your garden. If you go to the nursery and talk to them about what you want, you will probably have several options. You could conceivably buy an acorn, and plant it, grow it, and do essentially all the cultivation yourself. If the nursery sold you an acorn, it probably wouldn't cost very much. The next option would be to buy a seedling; more developed, but still small, and not worth a lot. Or you could buy a sapling, which would be worth more, or a well developed small oak tree, which would be worth

[79] 'Justifying the Rights of Pregnancy', p. 75.

quite a lot. It is logically possible (though probably not physically possible), that the nursery might sell you a full-grown tree, which would be worth a great deal of money (and would cost a small fortune to transport home to plant in your garden!). The greater the level of development of the oak, the more it is worth. In this case, the value is commercial, rather than intrinsic, but it does seem that the analogy can be applied to the case of the developing human.

It is important to remember the distinction between developing potential and mere potential however. Mere potential doesn't seem to make any moral difference, but developing potential does. This is not surprising, for developing potential is usually seen as more significant than mere potential, though it is also less significant than actuality. Consider the following examples. Every smoker is a potential non-smoker. But the person who is actively trying to quit smoking is developing that potential. Every criminal is a potential good citizen, but a criminal who is developing this potential deserves more respect from us than one who is not.[80] Every 17 year old is a potential licensed driver, but there is something significant in the 17 year old who is developing that potential by taking lessons.

To return to another example that we have already used, again suggested by Peter Singer, let us consider the case of Prince Charles and his potential to inherit the throne of England. This example seems to suggest that the nearer potential is to being realised, the more important that potential is. Prince Charles is not only a potential King of England, he is actually the next in line for the throne, and so the chance of him becoming King of England is quite high. The 50th in line for the throne (whoever that is) is also a potential King (or Queen) of England, in a way that I, personally, am not. But the potential of the 50th in line for the throne is so far from being realised that for all intents and purposes they have as much chance of becoming King as I do.[81] Thus while there is the potential for them to become King, it is so far from being realised that it is effectively non-existent.

If we apply this same sort of thinking to the question of foetal potential, then we arrive at a very interesting result. The newly fertilised ovum definitely has the potential to become a person. However, that potential is a very long way from being realised. The distance between potential and actualisation for the fertilised ovum has been graphically described by Bigelow and Pargetter in the following terms:

> The product of fertilisation is potentially a person. But the intrinsic changes during development are enormous. As the development takes place, the basis of the potentiality

---

[80] This example comes from Anthony Kwok-Wing Yeung, 'Mere Potential Persons and Developing Potential Persons'.

[81] Of course it is logically possible that they might become the King, while it is not logically possible that I should become the King, but the chance is so remote that it can be realistically left to the imaginations of fiction writers. See, for example, the 1991 Universal Pictures film, *King Ralph* (starring John Goodman), where every known heir to the throne is killed by an electrical fault during a royal photograph, and the throne eventually falls to an unemployed Las Vegas lounge singer.

of personhood continually changes. In the limit, at fertilisation, the product is potentially a person in virtue of potentially being a set of undifferentiated cells which is potentially a person in virtue of potentially being a differentiated foetus which is potentially a person in virtue of potentially being a highly developed foetus with functioning organs which is potentially a person in virtue of being potentially a baby which is potentially a person in virtue of being potentially an adult human being which is actually a person. Now while the potentiality seems to be transferred down this chain, we see no reason to believe that the value we place on the final categorical basis should be passed back up the chain, especially given the enormous change in the intrinsic properties of the actual as we move along the development chain. Thus we believe it is an error to assume that a value we place on a potentiality due to one kind of categorical basis must be the same as the value we place on that potentiality with a different categorical basis.[82]

While potentiality may grant some moral status to an entity, Singer is correct in suggesting that a potential-X does not have the rights of an X. Yet potentiality does seem to be capable of bringing about a change in moral status. It does seem to be the case that if that potential is close to being realised then the potential-X does have grants X a considerably higher moral status than a potential-X whose potentiality is far from being realised.

An opponent of this view might question what is actually meant by the phrase 'potential is closer to being realised', for there are several possible interpretations of the expression. It might, for example, mean that the realisation of potential is nearer in time. Or it might mean that there is a greater probability of the potential being realised, or that as it approaches the realisation of potential the being in question acquires more of the morally relevant properties. I would suggest that all of these things may be important, and that in the case of the developing human, all of these meanings amount to the same thing. As pregnancy continues, the realisation of potential becomes closer in time, there is a greater probability of the potential being realised, and the foetus acquires more of the morally relevant properties, such as sentience. Thus whichever meaning of 'potential being closer to realisation' is taken, the same conclusions about the moral status of the developing human can be drawn. The baby would have a greater moral status than the late-term foetus, the late-term foetus greater moral status than an early foetus, an early foetus greater moral status than a *conceptus*, and the *conceptus* would have greater moral status than the separated ovum and sperm.

However, it must be recognised that when the potential is an extremely long way from being realised, a small change in the potentiality status of the entity will probably have a negligible effect on its moral status. To return to our previous example, it doesn't really matter if one is the 50th in line for the English throne, or the 55th in line, the value of potentiality is so low in both cases that the resultant change in status can safely be ignored. This would suggest that the moral status of the embryo is very nearly the same as the moral status of the gametes that produce

---

[82] Bigelow and Pargetter, 'Morality, Potential Persons and Abortion', p. 178.

that embryo, and that the developing human does not acquire significant intrinsic moral status until some time well into pregnancy.

Chapter 7

Abortion and the Foetus as Non-Person

Now that I have made a detailed examination of the moral status of the embryo and foetus, I can return to the discussion of abortion and ectogenesis. I suggested earlier that the problem with severance abortion theories such as that proposed by Thomson, is that they do not reflect the desires of the women who actually seek abortions. Such women are seeking the death of the foetus, not merely its removal from their bodies. The distinction between decision responsibility and parental responsibility suggests that there might be some ethical alternative to parental responsibility, and since parental responsibility is not escaped by surrendering the child for adoption, the only remaining possibility for this ethical alternative would be abortion that includes the death of the foetus. But the death of the foetus could not be justified while at the same time granting the assumption that the foetus has the rights of a person. Thus it was necessary to examine the status of the developing human. Having concluded that the developing human does not have all the rights of a person, I return to the question of whether a woman is justified in demanding the death of the foetus as part of an abortion.

This is not a simple question to answer, for it may be the case that while the developing human does not possess all the rights of a person, that it does possess enough moral standing to preclude directly killing it. Mary Anne Warren, for example, has suggested that though an infant does not have the rights of a person, it is wrong to destroy an infant if people are willing to bear the emotional and financial cost of caring for it, since preserving its life does not violate anyone's rights.[1] Such an argument, as I have already mentioned, would apply equally to the aborted foetus if it was possible to preserve its life by transfer to an ectogenetic device. Thus the mere fact that the developing human does not possess all the rights of a person is not in and of itself sufficient to allow a woman to demand the death of that developing human in any abortion. Some further argument for allowing the direct death of the foetus will be required.

There are several arguments that can be made in favour of allowing the direct death of the foetus. The first that I will consider is the argument proposed by Steven Ross that the relationship between the parents and the foetus is of such significance that it is permissible for the parents to demand the death of the foetus as part of an abortion. Full consideration of this argument requires an

---

[1] 'On the Moral and Legal Status of Abortion', in R. Wasserstrom, (ed.), *Today's Moral Problems*, (New York: MacMillan, 1975), p. 136.

understanding of what is meant by the term 'good parent', so a lengthy digression into discussion of the meaning of this term will be required in order to fully assess Ross' argument. Another argument that I will consider is the suggestion that there exists a right not to be a parent. If such a right exists, then it could be used to ground a demand for the death of the foetus as part of an abortion.

After consideration of these arguments, I will also examine some other issues that are important in the context of abortion and ectogenesis, including abortion requested because of some defect in the foetus, and practical issues that would arise if ectogenesis was to be used as an alternative to traditional abortion.

Abortion and the Direct Death of the Foetus

Steven Ross is one writer who has argued that the woman's desire to see the foetus killed is justifiable.[2] In 'Abortion and the Death of the Foetus' Ross argues that most philosophical arguments about abortion are flawed because they do not take seriously the special status of the foetus. This special status is not due to any intrinsic properties, or to its potential, but is rather due to its special relationship with those people who will, if the foetus continues to develop, eventually become its parents.

Consider Thomson's argument for example. Ross points out that the problem with the argument is that the person on the other end of the kidney machine, the person who will die if we disconnect ourselves, is a complete stranger to us.[3] Now while the foetus is, in some ways, a stranger to us, if it continues to develop it will not remain a stranger. While there is no relationship with the foetus *now*, which makes it a stranger now, this will not be the case in the future. As Ross says:

> If we keep the violinist alive, our relationship to him more or less terminates the moment his dependency on us ends. We may get the odd invitation to concerts, but this is of a very different order from what we go through should we bring our child home.[4]

Thomson's argument fails, at least in part, because it fails to recognise the importance of the relationship between the mother and the foetus.[5] Even in cases of rape, where the analogy between pregnancy and the violinist seems to be the closest, due to the woman's lack of causal responsibility for the foetus' existence, the analogy still seems to lack something. Ross would suggest that what is lacking

---

[2] Steven Ross, 'Abortion and the Death of the Foetus', *Philosophy and Public Affairs*, 11 (1982), pp. 232–45.
[3] *Ibid.*, p. 235.
[4] *Ibid.*, p. 238.
[5] Thomson's argument may fail in other ways as well, but I am not concerned with that at this point.

is the acknowledgment of the future relationship that will exist if the woman decides to allow the pregnancy to continue.

Nor is it only pro-choice arguments that fail to take seriously this ongoing relationship. Ross also spends some time considering Herbenick's argument that elective abortion (that is, abortion for non-medical reasons) is like abandonment.[6] Herbenick suggests that abortion *is* early abandonment, because abandonment and elective abortion share the same features:

> The parent(s) (a) no longer wish to bestow their legal name upon the child in utero and once born; (b) no longer wish to retain the child in utero and, once born, as a legal heir to property; (c) no longer wish to provide support for the child in utero and, once born, as their own; and (d) no longer wish to retain any legal relationship to the child.[7]

Herbenick's suggestion is that once a woman signs consent for an elective abortion, there is evidence of her intent to abandon. At this point, the state could step in and assert its interest in redistribution 'on behalf of minorities denied the equal opportunity of parenthood'.[8]

Ross categorically rejects this interpretation of elective abortion as a complete misunderstanding of the motivation for seeking abortion:

> What (women seeking elective abortion) want is not to be saved from the 'inconvenience of pregnancy' or 'the task of raising a certain (existing) child'; what they want is *not to be parents*, that is, they do not want there to *be* a child they fail or succeed in raising. Far from this being 'exactly like' abandonment, they abort precisely to avoid being among those who later abandon.[9]

Ross points out that the special relationship parents have with the foetus is what makes the situation of abortion so different from any other situation. Whatever analogy is used to try to make sense of abortion ethics, it will fail in some way to account for that special relationship, which Mackenzie terms the acceptance of parental responsibility.[10]

Ross suggests that the foetus is unique, and that perhaps the best way to understand it is to draw on that uniqueness. Certainly the foetus has important intrinsic properties, but these intrinsic properties do not sufficiently define its nature for us to fully understand the range of emotions that the foetus may provoke. One of the properties possessed by the foetus, as I have argued before, is its potential to become a person. But merely seeing the foetus as a potential person is insufficient, for it does not explain the special concern that many parents have

---

[6] Raymond Herbenick, 'Remarks on Abortion, Abandonment and Adoption Opportunities', *Philosophy and Public Affairs*, 5 (1975), pp. 98–104, pp. 100–101.

[7] *Ibid.*, p. 102.

[8] *Ibid.*

[9] 'Abortion and the Death of the Foetus', p. 238 (emphasis in the original).

[10] Catriona MacKenzie, 'Abortion and Embodiment', *Australian Journal of Philosophy*, 70 (1992), pp. 136–55, p. 142.

for the foetus. Ross gestures here to Michael Tooley's example of the kitten that has been accidentally injected with a chemical which will cause it to become a person.[11] Tooley suggests that there would be nothing wrong with killing the kitten before the chemical takes effect, in other words, killing a potential person. But the foetus is more than simply a potential person. As Ross points out, 'it is potentially some particular person's *child*'.[12] Recognising this special relationship is the only way to understand the special care for, and interest in, a foetus that is taken by its parents.

Similarly, the desire to have the foetus dead is impossible to understand if only considering its intrinsic properties. Thomson suggests that if the violinist survives being disconnected from us, then we have no right to turn around and slit his throat.[13] But since the violinist is a stranger, the desire to have him dead is virtually incomprehensible. If someone other than a potential parent wished the foetus dead, then that desire would be equally incomprehensible. It is only the fact of the special relationship between the mother (and to a somewhat lesser extent, the father) and the foetus that allows understanding of the desire to see the life of the foetus ended:

> These two attitudes, being especially concerned for the welfare of the foetus and wanting it dead, which on the surface are so dissimilar, are in fact quite closely bound up with one another. Both stem from the same source: the fact that the foetus represents one of the potentially most central relationships possible to the one who carries it ... The foetus is the only thing that someone – a parent – may with equal comprehensibility and legitimacy care for or want dead.[14]

Ross suggests it is because the foetus represents such an important future relationship that it is understandable why a parent would care so much about it, and also why a parent would wish it dead. Either the parent values that relationship and wishes to have that relationship with this particular potential child, or they value that relationship and do not feel able to have the sort of relationship that they would like to have, with this particular potential child at this point in time. In other words, Ross suggests that, in many cases at least, the desire to be a good parent, and the understanding that one cannot be a good parent, are the motivating factors in the desire to have the foetus dead.

Given the importance that Ross places upon the desire to be a good parent, and upon the desire to make responsible parenting decisions, it is important to be very clear about what is meant by saying that someone is a good parent. Is it possible to

[11] 'Abortion and Infanticide', *Philosophy and Public Affairs*, 2 (1972), pp. 37–65, pp. 60–61.
[12] 'Abortion and the Death of the Foetus', p. 244.
[13] Judith Jarvis Thomson, 'A Defence of Abortion', *Philosophy and Public Affairs*, 1 (1971), pp. 47–66, reprinted in Richard Wasserstrom, (ed.), *Today's Moral Problems*, (New York: Macmillan, 1975) pp. 104–20, p. 119.
[14] Ross, 'Abortion and the Death of the Foetus', p. 236.

say that a good parent might make an ethical choice to kill the foetus that could become their child? In order to answer this question, I will have to make something of a detour, and examine what is meant by the term 'good parent' and what it is to make good parenting decisions.

What Does it Mean to be a Good Parent?

It is interesting that both Ross and Cannold discuss the idea of making abortion decisions based upon the desire to be a good parent, because it has been suggested that ectogenesis would actually allow people to become better parents. It is one of the arguments in favour of ectogenesis that is considered by Singer and Wells[15] and has been termed the *Better Parenting* argument[16]. This argument was originally suggested by Shulamith Firestone in *The Dialectic of Sex*.[17] She suggests that the development of ectogenesis would allow people to become better parents, as they would no longer feel the possessiveness that is experienced by many parents:

> A mother who undergoes a nine-month pregnancy is likely to feel that the product of all that pain and discomfort 'belongs' to her ('To think of what I went through to have you!'). But we want to destroy this possessiveness along with its cultural reinforcements so that ... children will be loved for their own sake.[18]

Singer and Wells suggest that this argument cannot be assessed until ectogenetic children are born, and James tends to agree with them. But I would suggest that simply dismissing such an argument is an inadequate response. Firestone suggests that the development of ectogenesis would make for better parents. While this is an argument that may not lend itself to direct refutation until we can actually compare parents of ectogenetic children and parents of children born through more traditional means, it is still possible to examine parenting, and see if the development of ectogenesis could plausibly make a difference to the practice. If it can not, then it would seem that Firestone's argument will fail.

Thus there are two reasons to examine what it is to be a good parent: first, to see if it is plausible to suggest that the desire to be a good parent might translate into a legitimate desire to see the foetus that-could-become-your-child killed, and second, to see if the development of ectogenesis could plausibly allow people to become better parents.

---

[15] Peter Singer and Deane Wells, *The Reproduction Revolution: New Ways of Making Babies*, (Oxford: Oxford University, 1984). Revised North American edition published as *Making Babies: The New Science and Ethics of Conception*, (New York: Scribners, 1985). The relevant chapter is Chapter 5 and is found at pp. 131–49 in the Oxford edition; pp. 116–34 in the Scribners edition.
[16] *Ibid.*, pp. 137–8.
[17] Shulamith Firestone, *The Dialectic of Sex*, (New York: Bantam, 1971).
[18] *Ibid.*, p. 263.

There are three possible senses of the term 'parent' which must be considered here. First, one can be a genetic parent. By this I mean simply that one contributes a gamete towards the development of a future individual. A man will become a biological parent by contributing sperm, a woman by contributing an egg. Second, one can be a gestational parent. By this I mean that one provides the environment in which the embryo and subsequent foetus develops. Usually this means a woman provides a uterus in which the foetus will develop, but it is also possible for the foetus to develop inside the abdominal cavity of both a woman[19] or a man.[20] Third, one can be a social parent. By this I mean that one has a strong emotional bond to the developing child after birth, and that this bond involves one in a nurturing relationship with the child.

In order to fully examine what it means to be a good parent, I would suggest that all aspects of parenting need to be considered. So I will consider the three forms of parenting in turn, and examine what it might mean in each case to be a good parent.

What might it mean to be a good genetic parent? Possibly the quality of genetic parenting can be determined by the quality of the genes that are passed on to one's descendants. This would make the good genetic parent equivalent to a stud horse. Or perhaps a man or woman who is extremely fertile might be described as a good genetic parent. Evidence for this fact might be that the woman frequently falls pregnant, or in the case of a man, that women frequently fall pregnant after intercourse with him. It would seem to me that the first suggestion here is the better one, and that parents who pass on good genetic traits are the most likely to by described as good genetic parents. So is this the aspect of parenting that Ross and Cannold have in mind? If being a good parent involves passing on good genes, then killing the foetus that will receive these genes would be a contradiction of the definition of a good genetic parent. The exception here might be where the foetus is aborted and killed because it becomes apparent that it is carrying defective genes of some kind. Thus it may be the case that a good genetic parent would see to it that a foetus would die under some circumstances. However, the cases that Ross and Cannold are discussing seem to be cases of elective abortion, rather than abortion due to foetal defect, so it does not seem that this is the sense of good parenting to which they are referring.

What about gestational parenting? What might it mean to be a good gestational parent? The most obvious answer would seem to be that a good gestational parent has little difficulty during pregnancy, and produces healthy babies at the end of the gestational period. It would seem that this cannot be the form of parenting that Ross and Cannold have in mind when they discuss the desire to be a good parent, for if it is possible for good parents to be doing the right thing in aborting and

[19] William A. Walters, 'The Artificial Induction of Abdominal Pregnancy', in *Bailliere's Clinical Obstetrics and Gynaecology: International Practice and Research – Human Reproduction: Current and Future Ethical Issues*, 5 (1991), pp. 731–41.
[20] *Ibid.*, pp. 739–40.

killing the foetuses, then obviously they are not talking about gestational parenting, since killing the foetus would contradict the definition of a good gestational parent.

What about social parenting? What does it mean to be a good social parent? Cannold provides an answer to this question, at least for the female parent. While the attributes of a good mother seem to be unattainable for any woman, at least this quote gives us an idea of what women think a good mother is:

> A 'good' mother is one who is always available to her children; she gives time and attention to them, listens to their problems and questions and guides them where necessary. She cares for them physically ... and emotionally by showing love. She is calm and patient, does not scream or yell or ... smack ... The cardinal sin of motherhood with its associated guilt is to lose one's temper with a child. Self control should be exercised at all times. Even in extenuating circumstances such as when a baby screams with colic for days or when the mother has no emotional or physical support in her task, she must at all times be in complete control of her emotions.[21]

While even God might have difficulty in attaining the standard described above, it does provide some idea of what a good parent is. Probably all, or at the very least, most of the ideals described in the quote could also be ascribed to the father.

Social parenting is clearly the aspect of parenting that Firestone has in mind when she suggests that ectogenesis might produce better parents, by removing the possessive feelings that parents have for their children. Improving the relationship between the parents and the child would seem to be a good way of improving the social aspect of parenting, but what evidence there is would seem to suggest that ectogenesis would not have this effect. If gestation is a bad thing, and produces possessive feelings that harm the relationship between parent and child, then it should be the case that parents who have not gestated would be better parents than those who have gestated. That would suggest that fathers should be better parents than mothers, since fathers do not gestate. In fact the opposite seems to be the case, since fathers are far more likely to abuse their children physically and sexually, seem to be more likely to abandon their children, and less likely to see their children after divorce. Thus the most obvious evidence available suggests that removing gestation will not improve parenting.

To return to the question posed by the writings of Ross and Cannold, is it plausible to think that women might seek abortion due to the desire to be a good social parent; or at least due to the desire to avoid being a bad social parent? In one sense this seems possible, for the common thought is that someone is only being a social parent after birth. If the child is never born, then one cannot be a good or bad social parent. Further reinforcement for this position comes from another quote supplied by Cannold:

---

[21] B. Wearing, *The Ideology of Motherhood: A Study of Sydney Suburban Mothers*, (Sydney: Allen & Unwin, 1984), p. 84, quoted in Cannold, *The Abortion Myth*, p. 88.

There is only one reason I've ever heard for having an abortion: the desire to be a good mother. Women have abortions because they are aware of the overwhelming responsibility of motherhood.[22]

When people talk about parenting, they are almost always talking about social parenting, so it is really no surprise that this is the aspect of parenting that Ross and Cannold discuss. It also seems to be the aspect of parenting that people place the most emphasis on, and consider to be the most important in cases where genetics and social parenting separate. Perhaps social parenting is the only *real* parenting, and is the only type of parenting that needs to be considered. Take the following case for example.

In this case a woman, Jane, and a man, Peter, have had an intermittent relationship for some time. Eventually Peter leaves Jane for another woman. Shortly after this Jane discovers that she is pregnant, and Peter is the father of the child. Before the child is born, Jane begins a relationship with another man, John. Eventually Jane gives birth to a baby girl, Gretchen. About a year after Gretchen's birth, Jane and John are married, and shortly after this, John formally adopts Gretchen as his daughter. Through all of this, Peter has no contact with Jane, John or Gretchen, although he knows that Gretchen has been born, and he knows that Gretchen is his child.

Let us consider the legal rights of these parents and see what insights arise from such consideration. Before I do this, there are some points of clarification that I must make. I am examining the legal rights that parents should have in such situations only because these legal rights give a good guide to the moral rights that the parents have. My invoking moral rights in this situation does not mean that I believe that rights theory is the only moral theory capable of dealing with such a situation, nor even that it is necessarily the best theory for dealing with such a situation. I do feel however, that invoking rights in such a situation allows us to grasp our intuitions about the case.

Suppose that years later, when Gretchen is eight, Peter tries to make contact with Gretchen, and over the objections of Jane and John attempts to assert parental rights to access and visitation, insisting that he is Gretchen's 'real' father, and that John is not. I think that given such a situation, most people's intuitions would be that John is Gretchen's 'real' father, and that Peter should not be able to assert any parental rights.[23]

The important question here is, why do our intuitions suggest this? Is it because John has formally adopted Gretchen? I think that the answer to this question is no. This is easily illustrated. Imagine that John had left Jane and Gretchen a few

---

[22] Dr Elizabeth Karlin, 'An Abortionist Credo', *Sunday New York Times*, 19 March 1995, p. 32, quoted in Cannold, *The Abortion Myth*, p. 87.

[23] In saying this, I mean only that the intuition is that Peter cannot assert rights over Gretchen. If Gretchen wishes to see Peter, or if there is evidence that it is in Gretchen's best interests to see Peter, then this is a different matter. In those cases what is being asserted is not Peter's rights, but rather a standard of the best interests of the child.

months after the formal adoption, and that no further contact had occurred between them. Then, at the same time that Peter re-appeared seeking to assert fatherly rights, John appeared also, and also attempted to assert fatherly rights. In this situation, the common intuition is that neither man really qualifies to be identified as Gretchen's father, and that the best description of her situation is that she is the child of a single parent family. If this is the case, then the formal adoption is shown to be essentially meaningless, in the same way that genetics are meaningless, without some other connection also existing. The only possibility for this connection is the relation of social parenting. In the original case where John lives with Jane and Gretchen throughout Gretchen's life, the common intuition is that he is the only one with a fatherly relationship with Gretchen, and that this is the most important criteria in this case, even if John had not formally adopted. I think this would be true, and that most people would agree. What seems to have occurred in this case, and what tends to drive people's intuitions, is that John has accepted the *responsibilities* of parenthood, and thus he can claim the *rights* of parenthood, since rights and responsibilities should, at least in the ideal, always go hand in hand.

A case like this one strongly suggests that social parenting is what is important, and that when we are talking about someone being a good parent, then we *must* be talking about them being a good social parent. In order to test this intuition further, it is necessary to examine some other cases with different features, and see if our intuitions always suggest that social parenting is the only important type of parenting.

Having considered a case where there was a somewhat accidental separation of genetic parenthood and social parenthood, let us consider a situation where that separation is quite deliberate, the case of insemination with donor sperm. In this case, let us assume that the rights of the mother are not in dispute. However, there are two fathers in this case who both have parenting connections; the sperm donor, who is a genetic parent, and the partner of the mother of the child, who will be a social parent. Both of these fathers have a parenting connection, so both of these fathers may have rights that ought to be respected in this case.

But the usual intuition is that this is not the case. When a child is conceived from sperm donation, most people have the intuition that the sperm donor has no rights with regard to the child, unless there is some further connection with the child as well, such as a social parenting connection after birth. This also seems to be the general intuition (though the intuition is not as strong) in cases where the genetic father has not been an anonymous sperm donor, but rather has been a party to conception in the normal way, through sexual intercourse. If there is no social connection after birth, then mere genetic connection to the child is not generally seen to be enough to assert any rights in the case. This has also been the prevailing view in American courts, where several cases have found that mere genetic connection is not enough for a father to assert rights to be consulted on the adoption of a child.[24]

We can also consider cases where a parent has a gestational connection, but no genetic one. Imagine a case where a couple wish to have a child, but while the woman has fertile eggs, she is unable to maintain a pregnancy. Suppose that one of the woman's eggs was fertilised with sperm from her partner, and then implanted into the uterus of another woman, a surrogate, to be carried to term. In this case, the surrogate mother has a gestational connection to the child she is carrying, but no genetic connection. If she was to give up the child to the commissioning couple after birth, she would have no social connection with the child. In a case like this, should the surrogate mother be able to assert any rights over the child?

Intuitions tend to be unclear on cases like this, especially when the surrogate mother attempts to assert rights immediately after birth when no social parenting connections have yet been established. If several years had passed before the surrogate attempted to invoke rights to see the child, then I think most people would agree that any rights that might have been able to be claimed would have lapsed. However, when the surrogate attempts to assert rights immediately following birth, then the situation seems to be somewhat different. At that time, the one person who has any sort of existing relationship with the child is the surrogate mother, and this seems to be a connection that is difficult to deny. However, when the courts in California were asked to rule on a case identical to this, the court ruled in favour of the genetic parents over the gestational mother, though the one female judge on the case dissented, stating that the court had not applied the usual rule of deciding in the best interests of the child.[25]

I think this selection of cases is revealing in two ways. First, they reveal the importance of social parenting, which seems intuitively to be the most important aspect of parenting in virtually all of these cases, probably because the acceptance of the role of social parenting carries with it responsibilities for the child. The few cases where our intuitions seem to be unclear are those cases where social parenting has not really commenced, and the issue of who has accepted responsibility for the child seems somewhat uncertain.

The second thing that is revealed by this selection of cases is another argument against Firestone's suggestion that ectogenesis might produce better parents. While discussing rights that might be asserted in various cases has revealed to us the importance of social parenthood, I think that it also reveals something else; the possessive nature of parental rights. This point was emphasised by Joan Mahoney:

> It seems clear from most of the decisions of the last several years in which courts have attempted to grapple with definitions of parenthood that they are getting it wrong

---

[24] See Joan Mahoney, 'Adoption as a Feminist Alternative to Reproductive Technology', pp. 37–9 in Joan C. Callahan (ed.), *Reproduction, Ethics and the Law*, (Bloomington: Indiana University, 1995), pp. 35–54.

[25] Gregory Pence, *Classic Cases in Medical Ethics*, 2nd ed., (New York: McGraw–Hill, 1995), p. 144.

because they are asking the wrong question. If one starts from the point of view of the parents and then tries to determine who has a 'right' to the child - to live with the child, make decisions about the child, determine who else gets to associate with the child - then parenthood cannot help looking like ownership ... given the multiplicity of family arrangements, the ownership model just doesn't help in determining parenthood, and it tends to lead to the commodification of children.[26]

If the problem that ectogenesis is supposed to solve, according to Firestone, is the possessive nature of parental relationships, then it would appear that the first thing that needs to be corrected is the ownership model of parenthood. When cases come before the courts, they are always decided on the basis of parental rights. As Mahoney indicates in the above quote, these rights tend to seem like property rights, and thus suggest that parents are 'owners' of the children over whom they assert these rights. Given this ownership model of rights, the predominant moral currency of our time, is it any wonder that parental relationships tend to be possessive. Compared to the overarching nature of rights-based claims, the problem of mothers feeling possessive about their children due to the pain of pregnancy and labour seems minor.

Social Parenting and Genetic Parenting

I have spent some time examining parenting, and have suggested that social parenting is the most important aspect of parenting, and that where there is a clash between social and genetic parenting (for example in custody disputes), that social parenting will take precedence. It has been suggested that the reality of our concept of the relative importance of genetic and social parenting is revealed in the term 'surrogate mother'.[27] Common usage of the terms 'surrogate' and 'mother' would suggest that the surrogate mother is the one who does *not* gestate the child, but rather is the one to whom the child is given after birth; yet the term 'surrogate mother' is used to describe the woman who gestates and delivers a child for another. The suggestion is that referring to the one who gestates as the surrogate occurs because the process of social parenting is seen as *real* parenting. Thus the woman who acts as the social mother is the *real* mother, and the woman who merely provides genetic and gestational factors is the surrogate.

Thus the cases that I have examined so far seem to suggest that good parenting is only about social parenting, and that there is nothing more to be considered. If that is true, then it would seem to be quite reasonable to suggest that the desire to be a good parent might lead a pregnant woman to choose abortion as a solution to an unwanted pregnancy. But there seems to be something missing from this story,

---

[26] Mahoney, 'Adoption as a Feminist Alternative', p. 43.

[27] See Hilde Lindemann Nelson and James Lindemann Nelson, 'Cutting Motherhood in Two: Some Suspicions Concerning Surrogacy', in Helen Bequaert Holmes and Laura M. Purdy, (eds), *Feminist Perspectives in Medical Ethics*, (Bloomington: Indiana University, 1992), pp. 257–65 (originally published in *Hypatia*, 4 (1989)).

because if social parenting is the only *real* parenting, then adoption would also be a viable solution for a good parent faced with an unwanted pregnancy, yet this option was universally rejected by the women who were interviewed by Cannold. That rejection of adoption suggests that there must be more to consider in thinking about what a good parent is. If one also considers the number of adopted children who seek out their birth parents, and the number of infertile couples who struggle to have 'their own' child through reproductive technologies like IVF, then the inescapable conclusion would be that genetic parenting does seem to be extremely important to many people. Consider the following case for example.[28]

In 1979, two couples, Ernest and Regina Twigg and Robert and Barbara Mays, both had daughters at approximately the same time in the same hospital. The children were mixed up at birth, with the result that the genetic daughter of the Mays (Arlena) was raised by the Twiggs, and the genetic daughter of the Twiggs (Kimberley) was raised by the Mays. Both families were struck by tragedy. Barbara Mays (Arlena's genetic mother, but Kimberley's social mother) died when Kimberley was 2, leaving Kimberley to be raised solely by Robert Mays (again, Arlena's genetic father but Kimberley's social father). Arlena Twigg died, at age nine, of a congenital heart defect, at which time blood tests revealed an inconsistency; further tests were undertaken that proved that Ernest and Regina Twigg could not be her genetic parents. When they discovered this fact, the Twiggs hired a private investigator to determine how this could have happened, and the hospital mix-up was discovered. The Twiggs eventually decided not to seek custody of Kimberley, on the condition that Robert Mays allow Kimberley to undergo genetic testing to determine whose biological daughter she was. These tests proved that she was, in fact, the Twiggs' biological daughter.

Who is Kimberley's real father in this case? Who is her real mother? A case like this seems to have no obvious answer. The importance that I have attached to social parenting would seem to suggest that Robert Mays is the real father, but that answer appears somewhat unsatisfactory in this case. Yet suggesting that those years of nurture are unimportant, and simply saying that Ernest Twigg is her real father also seems inappropriate. What should have been done if the Twiggs had wished to seek custody? A case like this can really only be answered by applying the usual legal standard of the best interests of the child, which in this case meant following Kimberley's wishes to stay with Robert Mays.

This case seems to throw doubt on my earlier assertion that social parenting is the most important aspect of parenting, for if that was so then surely there would be no question about what should happen to Kimberley. I would maintain that social parenting is the most important aspect of parenting, but the case focuses attention on the issue of genetic parenting. Other cases, like the Peter/John/ Gretchen case that I mentioned earlier, seem to suggest that mere genetics is not as important as social parenting: indeed I would suggest that it is impossible to be a

---

[28] Taken from Paul Lauritzen, *Pursuing Parenthood*, (Bloomington: Indiana University, 1993), pp. 76–8.

good parent unless one is a social parent, but the Kimberley Mays case seems to show that the genetic connection is also extremely important.

When genetic parenting and social parenting are deliberately separated, as is the case in adoption, there seems to be little doubt about what the most important parenting connection is, but most people still feel that an adoptee has a right to know who their genetic parents are. I would suggest that the reason that the Kimberley Mays case strains our intuitions is because her genetic and social parenting were *unintentionally* separated. I would also suggest that the reason that this is worrying is that there is a strong presumption that children should be raised by their genetic parents.

Consider the following facts. Courts are reluctant to remove children from the homes of their genetic parents, even when there is evidence that the children may be at risk of abuse. 'Best interests of the child' cases are usually decided on the basis of genetics in cases where two social parents compete for custody. Surrogacy contracts have been deemed unenforceable in many jurisdictions, because the rights of the genetic (and gestational) mother need to be respected: thus if she, as the genetic mother, wishes to raises her own genetic children, she should be allowed to. It is also clearly the case that genetic parents are not expected to give up their children simply because someone else might be able to provide for them better than the genetic parents can.[29]

A clear example of this fact arose recently, in the case of Elian Gonzalez, the six year old Cuban boy rescued off the coast of Florida.[30] Elian had left Cuba with his mother and a number of other people in a badly made boat, in an attempt to find asylum in the USA. The boat sank, and Elian was one of the few survivors. He immediately became the object of a custody battle between his Miami relatives (a great uncle and many cousins) who wished him to stay in Florida, and his father, Juan Gonzalez, who wished to have him returned to Cuba. Despite the fact that Elian's future was likely to be materially better if he stayed in the USA, and despite the fact that the people who wished him to stay were relatives (rather than strangers), the US Immigration and Naturalization Service (INS) ruled that Elian's father was the only person with legal authority to make decisions on his son's behalf, and ordered that Elian be reunited with his father. The INS in making its decision took into account not merely the genetic ties of father to son, but also the clear evidence of the social parenting of Juan to Elian. The INS ruling implicitly suggested that it was in Elian's best interests to be re-united with his father despite the fact that this would mean that Elian would return to Cuba.[31]

The women interviewed by Cannold, both those in favour of abortion rights and those opposed to them, also alluded to the expectation that genetic parents should

---

[29] This point is made in Gerald H. Paske, 'Sperm–Napping and the Right Not to Have a Child', *Australasian Journal of Philosophy*, 65 (1987), pp. 98–103, pp. 100–101.

[30] Details of the case are available from the CNN website; last accessed 15 December 2003. See www.cnn.com/2000/US/06/01/cuba.boy.05/.

[31] See 'INS Decision in the Elian Gonzalez Case', 5 January 2000, accessed 15 December 2003. Available at http://uscis.gov/graphics/publicaffairs/statements/Elian.htm.

become social parents. In interviews they often suggested that if they decided to adopt out their child, rather than aborting, there would be considerable social pressure on them to keep the child when it was born. For example, Gillian said:

> ... you can't hide away. I mean people will see you ... they'll assume that because you're having the baby you're keeping it ... You've still got to go to work ... go shopping ... see your friends. And they're going to assume you're having a baby because you want it, and not because you've made this moral decision that it's wrong to kill the baby ... So it's not only what you think, it's the pressures of people around you.[32]

The suggestion that children should be raised by their genetic parents has been made explicit in the academic literature on surrogacy. In their paper 'Cutting Motherhood in Two' Hilde and James Lindemann Nelson argue that bringing a child into the world exposes it to a risk of harm, and that the parents who are causally responsible for bringing that child into the world have a *prima facie* obligation to protect the child from that risk.[33] They further argue that since it is the child who holds the claim over both father and mother, the parents may not voluntarily relinquish the duty to protect the child.

Steven Ross addresses the issue in terms of the preferences of the pregnant woman.[34] Ross suggests that for many people there is a deep personal conviction about the way that they ought to live their lives, which includes the feeling that they, and not anyone else, ought to bring up any children they bring into the world:

> A woman may feel very strongly that she and not anyone else ought to raise whatever children she brings into the world. Or, more likely, that she ought to do so only in conjunction with a supportive husband who is also (and not by chance) the father of the child.[35]

While Ross recognises that for some people this desire is not so important and thus they might well be happy to give children up for adoption after birth, he suggests that this is not a view shared by many. Most people, according to Ross, see bearing and raising children as one of the most important tasks of their lives, and only want to do it in an environment they find right.

Summary – The Good Parent

So what can be concluded from this examination of what it is to be a good parent? It would seem that the conclusion is that our society believes that a good parent is a social parent, with a genetic (and if the parent is female, a gestational) connection

---

[32] 'Women's Response to Ectogenesis', p. 26.
[33] 'Cutting Motherhood in Two', p. 258.
[34] 'Abortion and the Death of the Foetus', pp. 240–41.
[35] *Ibid.*, p. 240.

to the child that they raise, and that while social parents without genetic connections can be good parents, genetic parents without social connections cannot. If a parent wants to be a good parent, then raising all the children that they bring into the world seems to be a necessity.

Given all of these factors, it would appear that the choices of a woman faced with an unwanted pregnancy are far more restricted than they might appear. If a good parent raises any children that they bring into the world, if becoming a genetic parent means that one ought to become a social parent, then most of the options available to an unexpectedly pregnant woman will be unacceptable. Adoption, in any form, including the foetal adoption offered by ectogenesis, would be an unacceptable alternative, as would any form of abortion that did not include the death of the foetus. The only acceptable options would seem to be a commitment to maternity, or an abortion that included the death of the foetus.

Abortion and the Direct Death of the Foetus Revisited

So after quite a long detour into discussions of what it means to be a good parent, we return to the question of whether abortion can legitimately include the direct death of the foetus, or whether the development of ectogenesis would mean that all abortions would become foetal evacuations. There are three central aspects that must be considered. One is the moral status of the foetus itself, which I have discussed at length in an earlier chapter. The second aspect is the responsibility of the parents for the foetus' existence. The third aspect is the relationship of the parents to the foetus. Before moving on to try to give an answer to this question, I will review the ways that the question *cannot* be answered.

Thomson's ingenious argument attempted to show that a woman has a right to an abortion even if the foetus is a person.[36] However, the right grounded by her argument is only a right to demand foetal evacuation, not foetal death. If an ectogenetic device could be used to save the life of the foetus, then according to Thomson's argument, its use would be required. Given the fact that the primary motivation in many abortions is to ensure that the foetus does not survive, the development of ectogenesis would frustrate that desire. While Thomson's argument may be used now to ground a right to an abortion that includes the death of the foetus as an indirect result, that would not be the case after the development of ectogenesis. Thomson attempted to circumvent the problem of whether or not the foetus is a person, but the development of ectogenesis would bring the question of foetal status back to the centre of the debate.

One of the main criticisms of Thomson's argument is that it takes no account of the causal responsibility of the woman for the existence of the foetus. Following MacKenzie, I would argue that where the women bears causal responsibility, this requires her to accept decision responsibility for the foetus, but that this does not

---

[36] 'A Defence of Abortion'.

necessarily commit her to motherhood. In cases where the woman is not causally responsible for the existence of the foetus, she has no moral responsibility for it, and an abortion can be justified by Thomson's argument. However, the only type of abortion that can be justified by Thomson's argument, even in rape cases and in other cases where the woman bears no causal responsibility, is foetal evacuation, not foetal death.

Mary Anne Warren has argued for a woman's right to an abortion at any time prior to birth on the grounds that granting any rights to the foetus would mean violating the rights of the pregnant woman.[37] In many cases allowing a woman an abortion would result in the death of the foetus. But again, the development of ectogenesis would change the situation, allowing the rights of the pregnant woman to be respected (at least to a degree) without ensuring the death of the foetus. While foetal evacuation may be a more invasive procedure than current vacuum aspiration methods of abortion, if the only basis for an abortion is respect for the right to bodily autonomy of the pregnant woman then I think that the current trends of protection of foetal rights would ensure that foetal evacuation would be required in all cases where the life of the foetus could be saved. Thus the development of ectogenesis would mean that the death of the foetus could not be assured in any abortion based on the right to bodily autonomy of the pregnant woman.

As I mentioned earlier, some arguments in favour of abortion will not be affected by the advent of ectogenesis. Arguments based on the lack of personhood of the foetus will be unaffected, and these arguments would allow a woman to demand the death of the foetus. However, I have also asserted that arguments like this are inadequate because they do not take seriously enough the potential personhood of the foetus, or the relationship of the foetus and its parents. Given that the foetus is a potential person, some special justification would appear to be necessary in order to kill it. Following Ross, I would argue that the special relationship that the foetus will have with the parents after birth if it is allowed to continue to develop provides that special justification.

Relationship and Foetal Value

I have argued earlier that the moral status of the foetus changes during pregnancy, with its moral status increasing as its potential for personhood increases. I have also argued that its intrinsic moral status early in pregnancy is very small. However, I do not think that this means that foetal value is small; foetal value is in many ways dependent upon the special relationship that it will have with its parents. In its early stages, the value of the foetus is almost entirely dependent upon the value that its parents place upon it. This reflects a suggestion made by MacKenzie:

[37] 'On the Moral and Legal Status of Abortion' and 'The Moral Significance of Birth'.

... although a foetus cannot be a bearer of full moral rights because ... it lacks the requisite intrinsic properties (namely personhood), nevertheless in a context in which some or more members of the moral community have decided to take parental responsibility for its future well-being, it has moral significance by virtue of its relations with her or them. We might say that in such a case it has *de facto* significance through her or them, until such a point when it can be considered a full moral being in its own right.[38]

If the parents highly value the could-be-child that is the early foetus, then its moral value is high because of the value that the parents place on it. If they do not value it, then its value is little more than its intrinsic value; that is, quite small.

Thus what I am arguing for here is a concept of foetal status where moral value is derived from a number of different sources. Some of the moral value of the foetus is derived from its intrinsic worth, which, I have argued, increases as the foetus develops. Some of the foetus' moral value comes from its extrinsic value to its parents as a future child. As the foetus develops, its intrinsic value assumes more and more importance in regard to its moral worth, with the extrinsic value becoming less important, until eventually, at a point somewhat after birth the child achieves full moral status, and the extrinsic value placed upon it by its parents ceases to make any difference to its moral worth.[39] I would suggest that the intrinsic value of the foetus is quite significant in later pregnancy, from about the time it develops the capacities of sentience; and that from this time on the parents rights to make decisions about its future will be limited, particularly in regard to demanding its death.

The idea that a being may gain moral status partly from intrinsic properties, and partly from extrinsic properties may seem unusual, but I would argue that it is a concept with which we are quite familiar. Consider for a moment the moral status of cats. Most people think that cats have some moral status by virtue of being a complex sentient creatures, and those people believe that it is wrong to needlessly inflict pain upon a cat. Thus there are laws intended to prevent cruelty to animals such as cats; people can be prosecuted for inflicting unnecessary pain upon animals; various organisations exist that seek to protect animals from unnecessary harm. However, since cats are not persons, they do not have the rights of persons, and most people do not think that it is wrong to kill a cat painlessly, provided that there is an acceptable reason to do so.

Yet *some* cats seem to have moral standing over and above that of other cats. If a cat is someone's pet, then it would seem that other people have an obligation not to harm that cat. Killing that particular cat painlessly would seem to be wrong in a way that killing a feral cat would not be. The particular cat that is someone's pet seems to have some moral status by virtue of being a complex sentient creature, but it also has additional moral status by virtue of the extrinsic value placed upon it

---

[38] 'Abortion and Embodiment', p. 143.
[39] *Ibid.*, pp. 147–50.

by its owner.[40] Thus it has moral status by virtue of two different factors, and the combination of these factors gives it higher status than either one of the factors alone could. An important corollary of this position is that if the owner of the cat wished to kill it painlessly (again, for good reason), that this would not be wrong. This also seems to be in accord with our intuitions. If, for example, a family is moving, cannot take their cat with them, and cannot find anyone else to look after their cat, there seems to be nothing intrinsically wrong in their having the cat put to sleep. Yet this same action, if performed by a third party without their permission would seem to be seriously wrong.[41]

A possible objection to this position would be that the cat is the property of its owner, and that it is the commercial value of the property that gives the cat greater moral status. This idea might explain the moral worth of the pure-bred show-quality Sphinx cat that cost its owner a couple of thousand dollars, but it certainly won't explain the moral worth of the family moggy that could be replaced for free at the local animal shelter. If the only additional value that is added by the ownership of the cat is the commercial value, then the family moggy would not seem to have any extra status at all, which certainly seems counter-intuitive.

The suggestion I am making here makes sense of some of our common intuitions about the status of embryos, foetuses and infants. I argued, when discussing the moral status of embryos and foetuses, that in some respects infants are treated differently from adults. The fact that non-treatment of newborns is even countenanced for conditions that would instantly be treated in adults, shows that they are accorded different moral status. The status that they have is nearly the same as adults, but it is clearly not the same. The decision to treat or not to treat in such cases will be made by the parents. If they value the infant, and in this particular case, the probable standard of life that infant will have later in life, then the infant will be treated. If they do not value the probable standard of life that the infant will have, then it will not be treated. Note that in both these cases the value that I am considering is the value of the standard of life that the infant will have, so it can quite clearly be the case that the decision whether to treat is made with the best interests of the future child uppermost in the minds of the parents. Thus the value that the parents places on its life, the extrinsic value, determines whether the infant will have the moral status of a person (and receive treatment), or a non-person (and not receive treatment).

Abortion cases are similar in many respects. The value that the parents (in this case primarily the mother) place on the life of the developing human, and the

---

[40] It could be argued that this is simply arguing that one should not kill someone's pet because of concern for the bad consequences, in this case the pain that it would cause the owner. However, I don't think that this makes a significant difference to the argument. The cat that is someone's pet still has de facto moral standing by virtue of the bad consequences that would flow from harming it.

[41] The ideas that I am articulating here are similar to the ideas proposed by Mary Anne Warren in her book, *Moral Status*, especially the 'Anti–Cruelty Principle', and the 'Interspecific Principle'.

future that developing human will have if it is allowed to continue to develop, determines whether or not it will be treated as a person, and allowed to continue to live and develop inside her uterus. Only the parents are justified in making such a decision; no one else can decide. This fact is pointed out by Steven Ross:

> ... if a psychopath could kill embryos *in utero* with a ray gun, we would not think this very far from murder. It is rarely noticed that only the parent's desire to see the foetus dead is ever taken seriously in the first place; no one else could possibly have a reason we would consider for a moment.[42]

This is similar to the cat analogy I offered a moment ago. The owner of the cat may make decisions about its future that no other person may make. While I don't believe that the parents of the developing human own it in the same way that someone owns a cat, I do think that there are sufficient similarities between the cases for it to be a useful analogy.

If what I have said so far is true, it would amount to a negative claim: that the parents do no wrong if they decide that they wish to kill the foetus, or have it killed. What would be more interesting would be if it was possible to make a positive claim, that the parents actually have a right to demand the death of the foetus. Such a claim has been made by Gerald Paske, in his 'Sperm-Napping and the Right Not to Have a Child'.[43]

The Right Not to be a Parent

Paske seeks to answer the question of whether a woman might demand the death of the foetus during an abortion. His reason for asking such a question is that he recognises that there is the possibility of developing 'in-vitro gestation' (that is, ectogenesis) which would mean that abortions could become foetal evacuations, rather than entailing foetal death. In order to answer this question, Paske uses the analogy of 'sperm-napping':

> A few weeks ago John was kidnapped and sedated. Several of his sperm were extracted while he was unconscious. He has now discovered that his sperm were used to artificially inseminate an ovum and that the embryo is being raised *in vitro*. (Assume that the embryo can be raised to viability *in vitro*.) The woman from whom the ovum was extracted has since died, and has left no relatives. The question to be considered concerns John's moral relationship with that embryo. What, if any, are his rights and responsibilities? Do they differ in any way from those of anyone else? If so, why?[44]

Paske uses the analogy of 'sperm-napping' because the idea of a man not having to gestate his children is more familiar than the idea of a woman not having to gestate

---

[42] 'Abortion and the Death of the Foetus', p. 244.
[43] *Australasian Journal of Philosophy*, 65 (1987), pp. 98–103.
[44] 'Sperm–Napping', p. 100.

her children. By creating such a scenario, Paske hopes to draw out intuitions about the case, and then apply them to the analogous female case, where a woman is being forced to become a mother (in this case a genetic mother), but does not have to gestate that child. Such a situation would be exactly what could occur in a pregnancy that results from rape, after the development of ectogenesis. The woman could of course demand that the foetus be removed from her body, but the foetus might then be transferred to an ectogenetic device, thus forcing her to become a genetic parent when she had no causal responsibility for the existence of the foetus. Paske wonders whether she might be able to demand the death of the foetus in such a case, and so he developed the 'sperm-napping' case in order to test intuitions about similar cases.

In his discussion, Paske recognises what he calls the 'fundamental value' of biological descendency in our society.[45] The idea of biological descent being a fundamental value leads Paske to make a claim very similar to one that I have already discussed, that children should wherever possible be raised by their genetic parents. Paske concludes that if John wished to raise the child that resulted from the sperm-napping, he should be allowed to do so, even if others also wished to raise it, since John is the genetic father of the child that will result from the sperm-napping.

More interesting is the discussion of whether John could demand that the embryo be destroyed, even though others wished to adopt it. Paske argues that in such a case opposing values must be weighed up: John's right not to have a child against the value of the embryo, the value of the consequences of preserving the embryo, and their combined value.[46] He assumes that the intrinsic value of the embryo is small, a position for which I have argued at some length, and thus suggests that John's right to autonomy is being weighed up against the good of providing a child to another childless person or couple:

> From John's perspective he is being asked to give away one of his future children on the grounds that (let us assume) this is the only way that an otherwise childless couple can come to have a child … John asserts strongly that he will do no such thing. Unless we are prepared to assert that fertile persons have an obligation to provide children for those who are infertile, John seems to have a plausible case.[47]

Paske believes that since the fertile do *not* have an obligation to provide children for the infertile, at least in this sort of society at this period in time, the conclusion must be that John has no obligation to give up his future child to someone else. Since he has no obligation to give up the child, and since the intrinsic value of the embryo itself is quite small, it would appear that John has the right to demand its death. Paske thus concludes that men who are the victims of 'sperm-napping' would have the right to demand an abortion that includes the death of the embryo,

---

[45] *Ibid.*, p. 101.
[46] *Ibid.*, p. 102.
[47] *Ibid.*

and analogously, that women who are pregnant as a result of rape also have the same right:

> They have this right not merely because they have the right to their own body. They also have the right to an abortion because they have the right not to have a child.[48]

Paske presumably uses the case of 'sperm-napping' and the case of rape as examples because he wishes to avoid muddying the water with questions of responsibility. But his argument would seem to justify far more than he allows. If the death of the foetus can be demanded in cases of rape, then it can obviously be demanded in all cases where the mother is not causally responsible (or not fully causally responsible) for the existence of the foetus, at least while its intrinsic value is small. Thus, following MacKenzie's account of causal responsibility, the death of the foetus could be demanded, at the very minimum, in first trimester abortions in cases of rape, incest, intercourse under duress, if the mother cannot be reasonably expected to foresee the consequences of her actions (for example, if she is mentally disabled, or under the age of consent) or in cases where the woman could not be said to be acting autonomously (such as if she was addicted to drugs at the time of the intercourse that resulted in pregnancy).[49]

The argument goes even further. In weighing up the right to autonomy of the parents, and the obligation to provide children for the childless, which does not seem to be a strong obligation at all, it would appear that the parents could demand the death of the embryo or foetus in all cases where the intrinsic value of the developing human is small. At the very least they could demand its death in all cases where conception was not the intended result of intercourse, since preventing the death of the foetus would force them to become parents against their will.[50] The conservative answer to this problem would be to suggest that a person does not have to become a parent if they become unintentionally pregnant, since they could always give the child up for adoption. But as I have already discussed in some detail, this is no answer at all, since our society has a strong presumption that genetic parents should become social parents, and many people have a strong desire to raise any children that they bring into the world. This being the case, the only way that the unintentionally pregnant woman can avoid becoming a parent is to seek an abortion that includes the death of the foetus.

[48] *Ibid.*, p. 103.
[49] See Mackenzie, 'Abortion and Embodiment', p. 138, especially note 5.
[50] Another writer who has suggested that a person should not be forced to accept parental responsibilities against their will is Michael Bayles. See *Reproductive Ethics*, (Englewood Cliffs: Prentice–Hall, 1984), p. 16. The suggestion that people should not be forced to assume parental responsibilities against their will arises in the context of discussing whether consent of the male partner should be required before a woman is allowed to proceed with artificial insemination.

In Vitro Fertilisation and the Right Not to be a Parent

The Tennessee case of *Davis* v *Davis* seems to confirm the view that people cannot be forced to become parents against their will. In this case, Junior Davis and Mary Sue Davis fought for custody of seven frozen embryos that were stored at the IVF clinic. Before their divorce, Junior and Mary Sue Davis had, apparently on many occasions, unsuccessfully attempted to have children through IVF. During the last attempt nine embryos had been created, two of which were inserted in the uterus of Mary Sue Davis, but pregnancy did not result from this attempt. Soon after the Davis' divorced, leaving the remaining seven embryos in storage. Initially Mary Sue Davis fought for custody of the embryos so that they could be implanted in her uterus; later, after her remarriage, she sought to donate them to another infertile couple. Junior Davis opposed both of these options, on the grounds that he did not want to be forced into becoming a father against his will. While the lower court ruled in favour of Mary Sue Davis, the Tennessee Supreme Court reversed this decision upon appeal.

Some of the arguments presented by Junior Davis in this case were especially interesting. He testified that he objected to Mary Sue Davis' use of the embryos because he did not want to be 'raped of [his] reproductive rights',[51] and after the lower court ruling he complained to the press that 'they are going to force me to become a father against my wishes'.[52] This use of feminist slogans and language in defence of male reproductive rights has incensed some feminist writers, notably Christine Overall. She argues that the vast difference in the consequences of the loss of reproductive freedom of men and women argue in favour of greater control over reproduction by women. In examining *Davis* v *Davis* for example, she compares what is required for both partners to produce the required gametes to create the embryos in the first place. On the one hand there is the emotional and physical ordeal of egg retrieval undergone by Mary Sue Davis, a process that does entail a degree of risk, and on the other hand, the simple and painless (and in all likelihood, pleasurable) process of masturbation for Junior Davis.[53] Overall suggests that this disparity in the cost of creating the embryos justifies giving Mary Sue Davis custody of them.[54] She further suggests that:

---

[51] *Davis* v *Davis* v *King* E–14496 (Fifth Ct. Tennessee), Young, Judge (1989) p. 21, quoted in Christine Overall, 'Frozen Embryos and "Father's Rights": Parenthood and Decision-Making in the Cryopreservation of Embryos', in Callahan, (ed.), *Reproduction, Ethics, and the Law*, pp. 178–98, p. 181.

[52] Ronald Smothers, 'Woman Given Custody in Embryo Case', *New York Times*, (22 September 1989), quoted in Overall, *ibid.*

[53] Masturbation is the most common way of obtaining sperm for use in reproductive technologies, but it is not the only way used. Some other methods of obtaining sperm from the man can be much more painful. I will discuss later some of the issues that may be raised by the use of these methods.

[54] 'Frozen Embryos and "Father's Rights"', pp. 187–8.

Men who want to control their sperm should be careful where they put it, and should pause to think before they provide their sperm for insemination or for in vitro fertilisation – even with women who are their partners.[55]

I think that Overall draws an unfortunate comparison between the intentions of an anonymous sperm donor and the intentions of Junior Davis. She suggests that since Mary Sue Davis is quite happy to raise any resulting children on her own, Junior Davis has no need to assume parental responsibility. The intent of an anonymous sperm donor is clearly to become a genetic parent and not a social parent. The intent of Junior Davis at the time of creation of the frozen embryos was to become a genetic and social parent of a child in partnership with his then wife. While it is plausible to suggest that Mary Sue Davis might be entitled to custody of the embryos if she wished to implant them in her own uterus, since this was the original intention in creating them, it seems reasonable to think that when Mary Sue Davis changed her mind and wished to donate the embryos, that Junior Davis' consent would be required. While some men may be quite happy to become genetic parents and have no social parenting connection with these children, other men are not. Surely that is the reason why not every man is willing to become a sperm donor. Junior Davis is among that group of men who feel strongly that children should be raised by their genetic parents. Since social parenting is not a responsibility that he wishes to assume at this time, he is seeking to prevent there being a child for whom he would feel the need to assume such responsibility. Thus his case, and his motivations, are essentially similar to the ones that we discussed earlier in our examination of the ideas of Steven Ross:

> What (women seeking elective abortion) want is not to be saved from the 'inconvenience of pregnancy' or 'the task of raising a certain (existing) child'; what they want is *not to be parents*, that is, they do not want there to *be* a child they fail or succeed in raising. Far from this being 'exactly like' abandonment, they abort precisely to avoid being among those who later abandon.[56]

The major difference in *Davis* v *Davis* is that it is the man, and not the woman, who is seeking to prevent the existence of a child that he will fail or succeed in raising. While normally it would not be possible to prevent the continuing development of an embryo after conception without severely violating the bodily integrity of a woman, in this instance the situation is rather different. If the embryos were located inside the uterus of Mary Sue Davis, then Junior Davis could only prevent their continued development by forcing her to have an abortion, which would be a massive, and totally unjustifiable invasion of her right to bodily autonomy. In this particular case though, the embryos are located in a freezer at an IVF clinic, and no one's bodily integrity need to be violated to prevent them from continuing to develop.

---

[55] *Ibid.*, p. 182.
[56] 'Abortion and the Death of the Foetus', p. 238 (emphasis in the original).

In fact, the situation here is remarkably similar to the situation that could exist if ectogenesis is developed. One genetic parent wishes to be a social parent, the other does not. Whose wishes should prevail? Overall considers three possibilities for control of the frozen embryos in the Davis case. First, she considers the possibility of joint custody, which she rejects on the grounds that this effectively gives the male partner veto, and gives unwarranted rights to what she terms 'ejaculatory fatherhood'.[57] Then she considers the possibility of granting custody to Junior Davis. She rejects this possibility also, on the grounds that either Junior Davis will employ a surrogate to gestate the embryos, which she considers to be extremely morally problematic, or that he will give them to a new partner to gestate. If he gives them to a new partner, then all the pain that Mary Sue Davis went through in providing the gametes will be used to benefit another woman: in other words, Mary Sue will be used as a means to an end, which Overall considers unjustified. Having rejected both joint custody and male custody, Overall concludes that only female custody is appropriate.[58]

But after the development of ectogenesis, it may well be possible for Junior Davis to gestate the embryos without any other woman being involved, since they could be carried to term in an ectogenetic machine. If this was to be the case, then Overall's arguments against male custody would seem to be invalid. The problem for Overall is that if this was to happen, then Mary Sue Davis' right not to be a parent would be violated, in exactly the same way that Junior Davis was arguing that his rights would be violated.[59]

It also seems problematic to place so much weight on the pain and emotional trauma of undergoing egg collection, since there is no reason to assume that the pain and emotional cost will always be borne by women in this way. Consider the following case for example. Let us imagine that a new procedure has been developed to deal with male infertility due to low sperm count. Men would be primed with hormones to stimulate extra sperm production, and then the testes exposed through surgery so that the sperm could be directly collected by aspiration. Such a procedure would be quite invasive, in much the same way that egg collection is now. If this had been the procedure that Junior Davis had gone through, then what would Overall say about the disposition of the frozen embryos? Both partners seem to have had an equal cost in producing the embryos; if custody was given to Mary Sue, and she donated them to another couple, then Junior's pain and emotional trauma would be used to benefit another man.

---

[57] The term 'ejaculatory fatherhood' was originally coined by Janice Raymond. See 'Of Ice and Men: The Big Chill over Women's Reproductive Rights', *Issues in Reproductive and Genetic Engineering: Journal of International Feminist Analysis*, 3 (1990), p. 49, quoted in Overall, 'Frozen Embryos and "Father's Rights"', p. 185.
[58] 'Frozen Embryos and "Father's Rights"', pp. 192–4.
[59] I should point out that since Overall sees abortion as a severance procedure, she may not be worried about the fact that women might be forced to become genetic parents against their will once ectogenesis is developed. I, however, am worried about this problem.

It seems to me that the only solution to such cases is to allow a modified form of joint custody. Overall complains that joint custody is effectively a male veto (apparently because women will always want to see frozen embryos raised and men will always want them to stay frozen!), but if and when ectogenesis is available, the force of this argument seems to be diminished. In cases where one party has had to endure much physical and emotional pain to create the embryos in the first place, it may be that it is appropriate to allow them to gestate and raise the embryos and the children they will become (by either natural or artificial means) since that would be in line with the original intention in creating the embryos. However, I would suggest that where embryo donation becomes an issue, that the consent of both parties be required, since no person should be forced to become a mere genetic parent without their consent, if it is possible to avoid this without violating the bodily autonomy of another.

Thus having examined this case, and the arguments of Paske, I would conclude that there is a right not to become a parent, but that right is not unlimited. The first limit on the right to not become a parent is the intrinsic value of the foetus: once it has reached a reasonable level of development, the right to demand its death will be severely limited. For example, I suggested that the foetus gains a significant measure of intrinsic value once it has achieved sentience. Does this mean that after the foetus gains the capacity for sentience the parents may no longer demand its death in any abortion? One thing that does need to be noted here is that not all foetuses develop at the same rate, so different foetuses might achieve sentience at slightly different times in pregnancy. Some severely disabled foetuses will never reach sentience at all (anencephalics for example) and thus it would be morally permissible to abort and kill such foetuses right up until the moment of birth, and quite possibly after birth as well. Thus it cannot be said with certainty that after a precise point in pregnancy ensuring the death of the foetus is impermissible. However, it does seem to be generally more problematic to demand the death of a more advanced foetus, and thus ensuring the death of the foetus will be more difficult to justify in later abortions. The second limit on the right to not become a parent is a due respect for the rights of others, most particularly for the rights of the other genetic parent involved in producing the embryo.

Abortion due to Foetal Defect

I now wish to turn my attention to another problem, the issue of abortion due to foetal defect. Of all the types of abortions this one is in many ways the most problematic, since abortion due to foetal defect is the one type of abortion where the death of the foetus is most clearly the desired outcome.

Prenatal diagnostic testing now makes it possible to detect a wide variety of foetal defects prior to birth, and the number of defects for which such tests are available is growing all the time. As many defects are now being detected early in gestation, parents know quite early in pregnancy about a range of problems that their future child has, or could have.

A decision to abort due to foetal defect is quite clearly a decision to prevent the coming into existence of a child whose prospects in life are poor. While it is possible to see this as a decision that benefits the future parents (for example, because it will save them the hardship of caring for a severely disabled child) I think it makes most sense to see this as a decision that is intended to benefit the future child. It is saying that the child would be better off not existing, than existing with whatever defect has been discovered. In cases like this, the death of the foetus is clearly what is intended in seeking an abortion, and not merely the divesting of responsibility for the foetus. The aim here is to end a life, not end a pregnancy.

This aim is recognised in many government programmes that fund prenatal testing. The assumption of many of these programmes is that abortion will follow if a major defect is found. In order to get funding for wide-scale testing programmes, health agencies often stress the cost-benefit that will be achieved. For example, researchers in Israel note that:

> The total cost of the program for the detection and prevention of birth defects for the fiscal year 1985/86 was approximately $370,000 ... Among the interrupted pregnancies there were 37 cases of Down syndrome. The calculated cost of their management was almost $5,000,000.[60]

Danish scientists agree:

> Prenatal chromosome investigation of women ≥ 35 years of age for Down syndrome alone would give a benefit of around ... $555,000 per year ... prenatal investigations are very attractive from the economic point of view.[61]

Prenatal diagnosis and abortion is only fiscally attractive for government if abortion entails the death of the foetus in such cases. If the foetus was to be transferred to an ectogenetic device and required long-term institutional care, which given the low adoption rates for disabled babies is quite likely, then the cost involved would be astronomical.

So it would appear that the death of the foetus is what is intended in abortion due to foetal defect. Certainly such an abortion may be fiscally advantageous for both the government and for the prospective parents, as well as being psychologically beneficial, but the interesting question is whether the abortion and the death of the foetus can be said to be of benefit to the future child. Does it make any sense to say that it is better off not existing than existing with some sort of disability?

[60] Juan Chemke and Avraham Steinberg, 'Ethics and Medical Genetics in Israel', in Dorothy C. Wertz and John C. Fletcher (eds), *Ethics and Human Genetics: A Cross–Cultural Perspective*, (Berlin: Springer–Verlag, 1989), pp. 271–84, pp. 274–5.
[61] Aage J. Therkelsen, Lars Bolund and Viggo Mortensen, 'Ethics and Medical Genetics in Denmark', in Wertz and Fletcher (eds), *Ethics and Human Genetics*, (1989), pp. 141–55, p. 146.

One writer who has attempted to answer this question is David Benatar. His strongest argument for this position is to suggest that people are *always* harmed by being brought into existence, whether they are disabled or not.[62] His argument is quite simple. If a person exists, they will experience both pleasure and pain. The presence of pleasure is good, the presence of pain is bad, thus the person who exists has both good and bad in their life. On the other hand, the person who never exists does not experience pain or pleasure. Not experiencing pain is good, even if there is no actual person who does not experience pain, and this is the reason that we think it is wrong to bring suffering people into existence. Not experiencing pleasure is not bad if there is nobody who is deprived of the pleasure. If we thought that it was a bad thing, then we would feel a duty to bring possible happy people into existence, and we do not feel such a duty. Thus the person who never exists is better of than the person who does exist, for there is good in both existing and not existing, but there is something bad about coming into existence, and nothing bad about never existing.[63] If this argument can be sustained, then it would seem that abortion that entails the death of the foetus can *always* be defended on the grounds that it is of benefit to the future child, provided of course that it takes place before a 'person' can be said to exist. However, Benatar's argument is controversial (to say the least) and defending it would take us some distance from our current topic.

Less controversial is Benatar's argument in 'The Wrong of Wrongful Life'.[64] In this paper, he examines the question of whether people can be said to be harmed if they are brought into existence with a disability, when the only alternative would be their non-existence. That is exactly the case with abortions due to foetal defect.

In discussing such cases, many philosophers have commented on the logical problem in suggesting that people are harmed by being brought into existence disabled, for the only alternative for such people is to never exist at all.[65] Certainly there are some cases where the life of the person who is brought into existence is so miserable and short that their life may appear, on balance, to not be worth living. Examples of such cases would include anencephaly, infants born without a digestive tract, and possibly Tay-Sachs disease (which leads to profound mental retardation and death before age five). However, most of the cases that we are discussing do not involve such severe disability, and the life that is likely to be led by these infants, if they are allowed to develop, is likely to be more pleasurable than painful. Can abortion and foetal death in such cases be said to be in the best interests of the disabled future child? Do such children have a life worth living?

Benatar's argument turns on a crucial ambiguity in the expression 'a life worth living'. He suggests that this term has two senses: a *present* life sense, and a *future*

---

[62] See Benatar, 'Why it is Better Never to Come into Existence', *American Philosophical Quarterly*, 34 (1997), pp. 345–55.

[63] *Ibid.*, p. 349.

[64] *American Philosophical Quarterly*, 37 (2000), pp. 175–83.

[65] For example, see Derek Parfit, *Reasons and Persons*, (Oxford: Oxford University, 1984), pp. 351–79.

life sense.[66] The *present* life sense of the term is synonymous with 'a life worth continuing', while the *future* life sense of the term is synonymous with 'a life worth bringing about'. These meanings are quite different, and it would be a mistake to apply the present life sense to future life cases. Thus while it may be true that a life not worth continuing is not worth bringing about (anencephaly might be a good example here), it is not true that a life worth continuing is always worth bringing about. Benatar presents the example of a person who is missing a limb. While few people would think that living life without a limb is so bad that such a life would be worth ending (thus life with a missing limb is worth continuing), most of the same people would think that it is better not to bring into existence somebody who lacks a limb (thus life with a missing limb is *not* worth bringing about).[67]

Whether a case is one of a life worth bringing about, or a case of a life worth continuing will thus be very important. How is the difference between such cases to be judged? In other words, when does a life start? I would suggest that this question needs to be answered in a moral, rather than a biological sense. Thus life in this sense starts not at conception, but rather when the foetus has significant moral standing, plausibly when it begins to have interests, at the point of sentience. However, a fairly strong argument could be mounted that a life does not begin in this sense until the acquisition of personhood. At the very least, for any 'life not worth bringing about', abortion due to foetal defect that includes the death of the foetus would be in the interests of the future child if carried out before the acquisition of sentience. For a 'life not worth continuing', abortion, including the death of the foetus, would *always* be in the interests of the future child.

Ectogenesis and the Right to an Abortion

A further important issue that must be considered when discussing the implications of the development of ectogenesis, is the question of whether the development of ectogenesis might lead to restrictions on the right to any sort of abortion. This question is considered by Frances Kamm, who suggests that there is a distinct possibility that the development of ectogenesis may well mean that some women might have no right to an abortion at all.[68] Kamm writes from the perspective of a deontologist, using Thomson's example of the violinist as the basis of her discussion. I have suggested that Thomson's argument is too restrictive, and that the right to abortion is broader than she suggests, but it is interesting to examine the problems that Kamm foresees.

Kamm refers to ectogenesis as External Means of Gestation, or Mechanical External Gestation (MEG). The two main types of MEG that she considers are

[66] 'The Wrong of Wrongful Life', p. 176.
[67] *Ibid.*
[68] See *Creation and Abortion: A Study in Moral and Legal Philosophy*, (New York: Oxford, 1992), pp. 208–18.

Partial External Gestation (PEG) and Total External Gestation (TEG). The difference between the two types is that a PEG pregnancy must begin in the womb before it can be transferred into a machine, while a TEG pregnancy starts in a machine and remains there for the entire pregnancy. In discussing the possibility of PEG, Kamm takes the same line as Thomson and Overall, suggesting that if the foetus could continue to live after an abortion by being transferred to a machine, then this is what is morally required. Kamm further suggests that if the machine can gestate better than a woman can, taking all factors into account, then a woman would be morally required to transfer the foetus into a gestational machine, rather than continuing the pregnancy herself. Of course, Kamm does argue, in a similar vein to James and Callahan, that if the removal procedure is more invasive and risky than a normal abortion, then the woman is entitled to a normal abortion.[69] Her suggestion is that the woman ought to try to save the foetus' life if she can, but that it is not necessary to do so if this would involve a significant cost for the woman.

Kamm's discussion of TEG is even more significant. She suggests that if the foetus cannot be transferred to a machine *after* gestation commences, but a machine is available *before* gestation commences, then this may well mean that the woman has no right to an abortion at all. Her suggestion is that if a woman has chosen to carry the foetus in her own body when an alternative that did not impose on her was available, then she has a duty to ensure that she performs the gestation as well as any available alternatives.[70] This argument assumes of course that the pregnancy was voluntary, but even so it suggests an extremely significant limitation of a woman's right to an abortion. To demonstrate the logic of the argument, Kamm returns to Thomson's violinist analogy. Suppose that a machine was developed that would help violinists with the rare kidney disorder that Thomson posited. An alternative to the machine is for the violinist to be connected to a person. Whichever method is used will need to be used for the next nine months, since it is impossible to transfer the violinist from the machine to a person, or from a person to a machine, without killing the violinist. If a person insists on being connected to the violinist, even though a machine is available, then it would seem plausible to suggest that the person must do the job as well as the machine. If the violinist's life could have been saved without the person's help, but they insisted on helping anyway, then it would seem unreasonable to allow the person to disconnect themselves, thus killing the violinist, when if they had not interfered the violinist would have survived.[71]

While this argument is in some respects quite reasonable, it does suffer from the usual problem of the violinist analogy, in that it ignores the special relationship that will ensue after birth. If the mother's situation was to change before the end of the pregnancy, then this would have a significant effect on her future relationship with the child, and may justify abortion. Such changes might include unforeseen

[69] *Ibid.*, pp. 214–6.
[70] *Ibid.*, pp. 216–7.
[71] *Ibid.*

medical complications in pregnancy, a severe change in financial circumstances or the death or disablement of a spouse. Any of these sorts of complications may have a severe effect on the environment in which the child is to be raised, thus making the mother unwilling to bring a child into the world at this time. Kamm's argument also fails to consider the possibility of a need for abortion due to foetal defect. The only cases in which her argument really seems to hold is in cases where a woman has voluntarily become pregnant, and then simply changes her mind about the pregnancy on a whim. I suspect that few women seek abortion for this reason, so Kamm's argument would only apply to a tiny percentage of women.

Ectogenesis and Economics: Considering the Bottom Line

An indirect, but significant, argument against the use of ectogenesis as an alternative to traditional abortion is the issue of cost. It has been estimated that there are about 1.5 million abortions performed each year in the USA alone. If the cost of ectogenesis is similar to the cost of intensive care for a newborn, which can easily run to over $100,000 USD, then the cost of caring, until birth, for all of the aborted foetuses that would now be placed in ectogenetic devices can easily be estimated. If only a third of the women currently aborting chose to use ectogenesis instead of abortion, then the cost in the USA each year would be in the region of $50 billion USD. David James points out that there would be a lack of adoptive parents for all of these children, and thus there would be a need for a huge number of orphanages and related services to care for them instead.[72] While the cost of ectogenesis may well come down in the medium to longer term, the expense in the short term would seem to make its widespread use as an alternative to abortion impractical.

There may be social costs that need to be considered as well, since there is some evidence that the legalisation of abortion, which includes the death of the foetus, has had a significant effect on crime rates in the USA.[73] In 'Legalised Abortion and Crime', John Donohue and Steven Levitt present three pieces of evidence that support this conclusion. One, there was a sharp drop in the crime rate in the USA in the 1990s roughly 20 years after the *Roe* v *Wade* decision. The peak ages for crime are roughly 18 to 24, so the crime rate declined at about the time that the first cohort affected by the legalisation of abortion would have been reaching their criminal prime.[74] Two, those states that legalised abortion before *Roe* v *Wade* experienced a drop in crime before the other states.[75] Three, those states where abortions were more frequent in the years following *Roe* v *Wade*

---

[72] 'Ectogenesis', p. 87.
[73] See John Donohue and Steven Levitt, 'Legalised Abortion and Crime', (1999) unpublished manuscript, available from the authors at Stanford University, and the University of Chicago.
[74] *Ibid.*, p. 3.
[75] *Ibid.*

(1973 to 76) show a substantially greater decrease in crime than in those states where abortions were less frequent.[76] Based on this evidence, and taking into account other factors that tend to influence crime rates, such as income, racial composition, and the level of incarceration, the authors of the study conclude that the legalisation of abortion can account for about half the recorded drop in crime rates in the 1990s. The authors also theorise that the reduction in crime rates is due to the fact that pregnancies that are most likely to produce a child who will grow up to commit crime, are also the pregnancies most likely to be aborted. This gives a reasonable explanation for the dramatic drop in crime rates, even though the legalisation of abortion had only a small effect on the overall birth rate.

If the authors conclusions are correct, then the costs of implementing ectogenesis as an alternative to traditional abortion are even higher than they appear, since ectogenesis would preserve the lives of all of these possible future criminals.[77] While such consequential arguments might have no strength if the developing human had the rights of a person from the moment of conception, I have argued that this is not the case, and such arguments do need to be taken into consideration.

Conclusions: Abortion and Ectogenesis

What conclusions can be drawn about abortion and ectogenesis from this discussion? Consider this quote from Deane Wells:

> In *The Reproduction Revolution* we say that with ectogenesis a termination of pregnancy would not imply the death of the foetus, so abortions would become early births, and we even say, somewhat whimsically 'Pro choice feminists and pro foetus right to lifers can then embrace in happy harmony' ... Ectogenesis is some years away ... I accept that the situation is likely to be less resolved than we may have made it sound in *The Reproduction Revolution*. In the abortion reconciliation argument we were really only trying to make the point that ectogenesis will create a great deal more common ground than had previously existed.[78]

---

[76] *Ibid.*

[77] In 1938, Dr Bourne performed an abortion on a 14 year old rape victim in Britain. He was charged, but acquitted, and the decision formed the basis of British abortion law to this day. One other doctor had already refused to perform the abortion, on the grounds that the girl could be carrying the future Prime Minister of England. See Cannold, *The Abortion Myth*, p. 7. The argument that abortion might deprive the world of a great leader/scientist/ doctor/artist is a common argument presented by opponents of abortion, but the evidence presented by Donohue and Levitt suggests that it is more likely that abortion will deprive the world of a future serial killer!

[78] Deane Wells, 'Ectogenesis, Justice and Utility: A Reply to James', *Bioethic*, 4 (1987), pp. 372–9, pp. 377–8. Included quote from *The Reproduction Revolution*, p. 135.

I would suggest that Wells is wrong in nearly every respect. The development of ectogenesis would not resolve anything at all and would not create any common ground; it merely shifts the focus of the debate back from the grounds of a woman's right to control her body to the older grounds of the moral status of the foetus.

Both pro-choice and anti-choice activists seem to agree that a good parent raises any children that they bring into the world. Thus when faced with an unwanted pregnancy, for the woman who wishes to be a good parent there are only two choices: abortion including foetal death, or motherhood. The development of ectogenesis does not reconcile this problem, since it preserves the life of the foetus. If a good parent raises any children they bring into the world, then a good parent would not choose ectogenesis as a solution to an unwanted pregnancy.

Thus in most cases where an abortion is being performed and the mother has decided not to assume parental responsibility, the advent of ectogenesis will not be welcomed, if this results in a denial of the women's ability to demand the death of the foetus. In discussing the interviews of Cannold, I noted that the pro-choice women felt that the death of the foetus was an integral part of an abortion. The purpose of abortion in such cases is not to evict the foetus from the uterus, as one might evict a tenant from a house. Rather it is to prevent the existence of a being for whom the woman would in future be responsible; even if she was only responsible in a genetic sense. Since a good parent, especially a good mother, raises any children that they have brought into existence, the only way to deal with an unwanted pregnancy when one does not feel able to assume parental responsibility is to ensure that there is not a child brought into existence. To use the words of Steven Ross:

> As many antiabortionists say now, and doubtless many more would say given the possibility of abortion₁ (ectogenesis), you don't have to bring it home, you could very well abandon it and put it up for adoption ... But this course of action would not stop our being parents, at least not in one rather obvious sense of the term. It would not in fact free our life of a certain kind of complication. Although we would not be bringing the child up, because someone else ... is all too gladly embracing those tasks, we do not want precisely this state of affairs to come about.[79]

Ectogenesis allows one to become a genetic parent without having to be a social parent or a gestational parent, but this is exactly the state of affairs that these women wish to avoid. If they become genetic parents, they believe that becoming social parents is a non-negotiable consequence. Thus they wish not to become genetic parents, by ensuring that the embryo or foetus that is currently developing ceases to develop. If the development of ectogenesis meant that they were no

---

[79] Ross, 'Abortion and the Death of the Foetus', pp. 138–9. My insert. The abortion₁ to which Ross refers is abortion that does not entail the death of the foetus, in other words, ectogenesis.

longer free to choose the death of the foetus, then these women would certainly not welcome its development.

On the other hand, in cases where there is a positive desire to parent, and an abortion is indicated for maternal medical reasons, the development of ectogenesis would probably be welcomed. In such cases the desire is not to prevent the existence of a future child, but rather to prevent health problems for the mother. In other words, there genuinely are cases where the desire is the desire to end the pregnancy, not to kill the foetus. Many women who seek abortions for medical reasons would be delighted if the life of the foetus could be saved. For example, Singer and Wells cite the case of Toby and Isabel Bainbridge, who were early patients in one of the IVF programmes in Melbourne. IVF failed to help them to have a child, and eventually they decided to stop trying, by which time Isabel had been attempting to become pregnant, by one method or another, for 17 years. However, during this period, Isabel Bainbridge had become pregnant on two occasions. Both of these pregnancies had been ectopic pregnancies, where the embryo had begun to develop in a fallopian tube rather than the uterus, and both of these pregnancies had to be aborted to protect Isabel's life.[80] If ectogenesis had been available in these cases, the embryo could have been transferred to an ectogenetic device, the risk to Isabel's life would have been ended, and she would still have had a child. Similarly, Lesley Brown, mother of the first IVF child Louise Brown, had also had previous ectopic pregnancies, which had to be aborted.[81]

For most women seeking abortion, the aim is not simply to end the pregnancy, but to end the life of the foetus. I would suggest that not only do women do nothing wrong in seeking to end the life of the foetus, but in most cases they actually have the right to demand foetal death. This is because the moral status of the foetus is so intimately connected to the present and future relationship it has with its parents. They, and only they, are entitled to make decisions about its future.

Other reasons for thinking that the development of ectogenesis would cause more problems than it would solve with regard to abortion include the possibility that it could be used to restrict the availability of any type of abortion, and the massive costs that would be involved in implementing any programme of ectogenetic (that is, evacuative) abortions.

Overall it would seem that the development of ectogenesis would not bring any resolution to the abortion debate. It would have the effect of focussing the debate onto the areas of real conflict, but it would not afford pro-choice feminists and pro-foetus right to lifers any more opportunity to embrace in happy harmony than they have already.

---

[80] *The Reproduction Revolution*, pp. 20–22.
[81] See Pence, *Classic Cases*, pp. 96–7.

Chapter 8

The Developing Human as a Source of Donor Organs

It might well be the case that if ectogenetic technology was to be developed, that it would have no effect whatsoever on the abortion debate. The development of ectogenesis will only really be important for abortion if the technology can be used to continue a pregnancy that has begun in the uterus. If the technology was to be developed in such a way that it could only be used from before conception, then the only effect that this could have on the abortion debate would be the possibility that this might lead to some restrictions on the right to an abortion where pregnancy was the intended result of intercourse. This is a possibility suggested by Frances Kamm,[1] that I discussed in the previous chapter. However, even if the technology can only be used for new pregnancies, there will still be important ethical implications for its use. First, it could be used as another reproductive technology to aid the infertile, mainly as a substitute for surrogacy, but also for other women for whom pregnancy is likely to be dangerous. This possibility was discussed in some detail in the objections to ectogenesis. But ectogenetic technology might not only be used as a replacement for surrogacy. There are also important possibilities for the use of ectogenesis in the area of transplant surgery.

Modern medicine uses tissue and organ transplants in a large number of ways, and scientific advances continually increase these options. For example, cornea and kidney transplants are a daily occurrence, and heart or heart-lung transplants take place frequently. At present there are two major problems with such transplants. The first problem with transplants is the lack of suitable donor organs. Most organ donations can only come from corpses,[2] and many corpses are not suitable as donors in any case, for various reasons. A person who dies of congestive heart failure for example, is certainly not going to be a good candidate for providing a donor heart. Even fewer of the suitable donor corpses can actually be used, as consent for organ donation is frequently hard to obtain.

The second problem with transplants is the likelihood of organ rejection. Unless the donor is closely related to the recipient, it is likely that the immune

[1] See *Creation and Abortion*, (Oxford: Oxford University, 1992), pp. 208–220.
[2] By 'corpse' I mean someone who is categorised as dead by whatever local laws apply. Most organs suitable for transplant come from those who are classified as brain dead, but whose hearts are still beating.

system of the recipient will attack the donor organ or tissue as if it was a foreign body. Immuno-suppressent drugs can help to alleviate this problem, but they have their own side-effects. The risk of rejection varies with the type of transplant, and in some cases is so high that the only way to overcome the problem is to use tissue from an identical twin. Since identical twins are rare, few people are able to benefit from some types of transplants.

The use of embryos and foetuses could overcome these problems. If the embryos were to be specially grown for the purpose of organ or tissue donation, then this would overcome the problem of the scarcity of suitable donors. Embryonic tissue also seems to be less prone to rejection than adult tissue. However, the problem of rejection could be solved in an even more dramatic way. Now that mammalian cloning has become a reality, it is theoretically possible that scientists would be able to create a clone of the recipient, and grow that clone through ectogenesis. Any tissues or organs removed from this clone would be genetically identical to those of the recipient – everyone could have an identical twin to donate organs for them.

Now it may seem that any organs or tissues produced by this method would be too small to be of any use, except for other infants. This would still be a significant gain from the present time, since organs for donation to infants are in especially short supply. However, it may well be the case that the use of such organs would not be limited merely to infants. If the embryo were to be kept alive until the organs had begun to form, then it may be possible to remove those organs, and place then in a special culture that would rapidly grow them to adult size.

Partial Ectogenesis for Transplant

Writers such as Singer and Wells have suggested that a strong argument for pursuing ectogenetic research could be advanced on the basis that it would enable partial ectogenesis for transplant purposes.[3] Using ectogenetic techniques in this way would increase the supply of donor organs by providing numbers of embryos from which organs could be harvested. Coupling ectogenesis with further developments in the area of cloning might well mean that every person would have access to compatible organs for transplantation, provided there was time to grow the required organs. As Singer and Wells point out, this whole procedure would not be complete ectogenesis, but merely partial ectogenesis, since the embryo would not be brought to a point where it would be able to survive on its own. 'Its survival is not the point of the procedure; the survival of others is.'[4]

---

[3] Peter Singer and Deane Wells, *The Reproduction Revolution: New Ways of Making Babies*, (Oxford: Oxford University, 1984), pp. 138–9.
[4] Singer and Wells, *The Reproduction Revolution*, p. 139.

Singer and Wells are quite clear that if one was to grow embryos to farm them for organs, then the embryos would need to be killed before there was any chance of them experiencing pain:

> If there is any suspicion that an embryo has developed the rudiments of a brain, or that it has become sentient, then it is too late for it to be used for any sort of transplant surgery or research. There must always be a safety margin. No being – of any species – deserves to have gratuitous pain inflicted upon it.[5]

Singer and Wells do consider another possibility here, that one might keep an embryo alive longer than this, but only after an operation that destroyed any chance of the embryo ever attaining consciousness. If such an operation was performed on a growing foetus before it was capable of feeling pain, this would seem to place this embryo in the same ethical category as a brain dead adult. It would be incapable of any conscious experience yet able to be kept alive by artificial means until organs were ready for harvesting. After all, if it is permissible to create an embryo for the purpose of producing organs for transplantation, and then kill that embryo before it ever attains consciousness, then what possible difference could it make to the embryo itself if the possibility of consciousness were removed, yet the embryo was kept alive for a longer period?[6]

On such a proposal Singer and Wells urge caution. While they agree that if all feelings are put aside, there is no difference between a pre-sentient embryo and one whose capacity for sentience has been removed, they also think that it is almost impossible to actually set those feelings aside. They suggest that our feelings of care and protection for infants run very deep, and that for the sake of all children those feelings should not be imperilled. If creating non-sentient infants as organ donors would damage the instinct to protect sentient infants, then creating such non-sentient infants should be avoided. It should be noted that Singer and Wells do not see any direct wrong in such a procedure: the wrong caused would be a side effect; the damage caused to our society.

James criticises Singer and Wells on this point, and suggests that they are being inconsistent as utilitarians.[7] I do feel that James has missed the point somewhat, for he states that Singer and Wells reject the partial ectogenesis for transplant argument entirely, whereas they have actually only rejected one facet of the argument. Singer and Wells agree with not allowing embryos to grow to the stage where they are sensate if their organs are to be used for transplantation, but they certainly do not reject the argument as a whole. In any case, I see no difficulty with preference utilitarians such as Singer and Wells rejecting this portion of the argument. If most preferences would be satisfied by *not* creating damaged infants for organ farming, then surely that is the course of action that a preference utilitarian would want to follow.

[5] *Ibid.*, p. 148.
[6] *Ibid.*
[7] James, 'Ectogenesis', pp. 83–6.

But what of the whole argument? Singer and Wells reject a portion of the ectogenesis for transplant argument, but they certainly do not reject the whole thing. If ectogenesis were to be developed, then Singer and Wells would be committed to using the technology to grow embryos and foetuses for use in transplant surgery. This leads me to consider whether ectogenetic technology should be used to create embryos that would be used to provide organs for transplant surgery, with the proviso that any organs would be removed before the resulting foetus had the capacity to feel pain. A simple, but probably inadequate answer, would be to again rely on preference utilitarianism. If most people have a preference that ectogenesis should not be used to create organs for transplant surgery, then this is the course of action that should be followed.

I suspect that is actually the case, and that most people would be opposed to the idea of farming foetal parts in this way. However, there is not a great deal of hard evidence that I can present for this position. The grimaces of disgust that most people have given me when I have brought up the topic might be considered to be evidence (the YUK! reaction in play once again) but this is hardly scientific. Perhaps the number of people who are opposed to abortion generally, or will only allow abortion to safeguard the life of the mother, might also be considered to be evidence of general opposition to killing the foetus for the purposes of organ donation. But again, it is hard to quantify this. Without some broad-based non-partisan discussion of the topic, it is hard to see any way of accurately determining people's preferences on this issue. In order to decide if it is appropriate to use ectogenesis in this way, it will be necessary to seek some other arguments on the topic. This is likely to provide the most satisfactory answer in any case, since most people are not preference utilitarians, so an answer founded on that theory is unlikely to win broad support.

So let me ask the question once again: Should we should use ectogenetic technology to create embryos that would be used to provide organs for transplant surgery? This is not yet a widely discussed topic. The publicity over cloning has led to some discussion of the ethics of cloning people to provide organs for transplantation, but such discussion has been mainly confined to the popular press and internet chat sites, rather than the academic literature. As any child produced by cloning at present would have to be carried in the uterus of a woman, in order for its organs to be used for transplant purposes it would have to either be aborted or killed after birth. Since killing the cloned child after birth would be murder, this does tend to limit discussions of the usefulness of cloned beings for transplant purposes to those organs that are paired in the body, kidneys for example, rather than to discussing the use of all bodily organs. The use of tissues or organs from aborted cloned foetuses has not been discussed at all.

However, there has been some discussion of the issue of using non-cloned foetal tissues for transplant purposes. Such tissues are obtained after spontaneous or induced abortion of pregnancy, and thus may come from foetuses at varying stages of development. The ethical issues regarding the use of such foetal tissues have similarities with the issues under discussion, and highlight some important issues. Therefore, I will now turn my attention to discussions of the use of foetal tissues in research and treatment.

One issue that arises in the case of usage of foetal tissues is the fact that most foetal tissues that are available for use have come from induced, rather than spontaneous abortions.[8] Thus some people feel that the tissues are in a way morally tainted by their origins, and that they should not be used in any subsequent experiments or treatments. Such a view is usually based on an ethical theory that either opposes abortion outright, or presumes that the only grounds for justifying an abortion is the right to bodily autonomy of the mother. I have already argued against such views in suggesting that the parents of the foetus, in particular its mother, may have the right to demand the death of the foetus, so I will not discuss them further here. This particular issue would not arise in the case of partial ectogenesis for transplant, since such a procedure already assumes that abortion, including the death of the foetus, can be justified on some grounds other than that of the bodily autonomy of the mother. If the foetus cannot be killed except to preserve the bodily autonomy of the mother, then partial ectogenesis for transplant need not even be considered. Thus to even consider this an option means basing the abortion decision on a theory that allows abortion on other grounds. Ethical theories that allow abortion on other grounds will not (generally) consider tissues obtained from an abortion to be 'tainted' by the mere fact of abortion. If there are moral problems involved in the use of foetal tissues, then they would arise from more than the mere fact of abortion.

The use of foetal tissues in research and treatment was an issue in the United Kingdom in the mid-1980s, and was referred to a Government appointed committee for consideration. This Committee to Review the Guidance on the Research Use of Foetuses and Foetal Material (FFMC) reported in July 1989. The Code of Practice which they suggested, also referred to as the Polkinghorne Report, has been used as a guide in many jurisdictions, and so is worthy of some consideration, especially in regard to its conditions for the use of foetal material. In examining this Code, I will draw heavily on the discussion of John Polkinghorne, chairman of the FFMC.[9]

FFMC Code of Practice

The FFMC Code of Practice places two main conditions on the use of foetal tissue. First, the Code insists that there is a clear separation between the act of abortion and any subsequent use of foetal materials. In order to achieve this separation, the FFMC recommended the establishment of a government funded tissue bank to act

---

[8] For example, at one 'Foetal Tissue Bank', foetuses from spontaneous abortions made up between 0.2 and 0.3 per cent of the available foetuses for the supply of tissues. See Peter McCullagh, *The Foetus as Transplant Donor: Scientific, Social and Ethical Perspectives*, (Chichester: John Wiley & Sons, 1987), p. 193.

[9] J. C. Polkinghorne, 'Law and Ethics of Transplanting Foetal Tissue' in Robert G. Edwards, (ed.), *Foetal Tissue Transplants in Medicine*, (Cambridge: Cambridge University, 1992), pp. 323–335.

as an intermediary between the source of the foetal tissue, and the user of that tissue (for the purposes of research, treatment and so on). The second condition placed on the use of foetal tissue is the demand that the informed consent of the mother be obtained before the use of any tissues. Given the fact of the earlier insistence on the separation of the source and user of foetal materials, the consent given can only be consent in the most general terms, and must be separate from, and subsequent to, the consent to the actual abortion.

The reason for insisting upon separation of the abortion decision from any subsequent use of foetal tissues was to eliminate (as far as humanly possible) some of the possible unwanted side effects of allowing the use of foetal tissues obtained from abortions. These unwanted effects include such things as pressure being placed upon women to abort in order to allow the abortion provider themselves to research particular problems using foetal tissue.[10] Another possibility is that women who have particular conditions that may prove interesting might be pressured to abort to see if these conditions affect the foetus as well.[11] Another unwanted effect is what was known to the FFMC as 'targeting', deliberately generating foetuses to provide material for some particular purpose or individual need.[12] Yet another possibility that the FFMC wished to avoid was the use of foetal ovarian tissue to enable women with no ovaries to conceive.[13] Having mentioned these particular problems, I would now like to briefly discuss each of them and see why the FFMC considered such practices to be unethical, and thus why they established the particular conditions for the use of foetal material that they laid out in the Code of Practice.

The FFMC decided that it was not necessary to answer questions such as whether the foetus is a person, or when it can be considered to be alive, or human and so on. Rather they followed the lead of the Warnock Committee, and answered the different question 'How is it right to treat the human embryo (and foetus)?'[14] The FFMC decided that 'On the basis of its potential to develop into a human being, a foetus is entitled to respect, according it a status broadly comparable to that of a living person'.[15] Given this particular view of the status of the embryo and foetus, the FFMC concluded that there were only two morally relevant categories of foetus; alive or dead,[16] and thus that:

> A living foetus should be treated on principles broadly comparable to those applicable to children and adults: no intervention above minimal risk except on balance for the benefit

---

[10] *Ibid.*, p. 327.

[11] *Ibid.*

[12] *Ibid.*, p. 328.

[13] *Ibid.*

[14] From the report of the Warnock Committee, paragraph 11.9, quoted in Polkinghorne, 'Law and Ethics of Transplanting Foetal Tissue', *ibid.*, p. 325, my insert.

[15] FFMC report paragraph 9.1, quoted in Polkinghorne, 'Law and Ethics of Transplanting Foetal Tissue', *ibid.*

[16] *Ibid.*

of the foetus. The only exception relates to termination of pregnancy under the Abortion Act (1967), in which case ethical considerations relating to the welfare of the mother come into play.[17]

The Abortion Act depends upon the 'necessity' defence, which means that the act specifically enshrines the doctor's role as gatekeeper, and thus makes it the duty of the doctor to ensure that women do not get abortions on demand, but only when the doctor feels it is medically necessary. In order for an abortion to be legal, a doctor who has performed an abortion must be able to prove that they sincerely believed that the abortion was necessary to safeguard the welfare of the patient.[18]

Obviously there is a great deal that could be said about the particular definition of moral status that the FFMC has used, and shortly I will consider objections to, and the various problems with, this position. First, though, I wish to simply accept the FFMC's position. Given this particular definition and understanding of the moral status of the foetus, it is easy to see why the FFMC was worried about a pregnant woman being pressured to abort in order to provide foetal tissue. Women in the United Kingdom do not have a right to abortion, it is only legal when it is necessary to safeguard the women's health, broadly construed. Pressure placed on a woman to induce her to abort might have a significant effect upon her mental state, and may even make an abortion necessary where previously it was not necessary. If this was to be the case, then the abortion would become legal where it would previously have been illegal. Given these sorts of issues, it is quite easy to understand why the FFMC insisted upon separation of the abortion decision from the decision to allow use of any foetal tissues.[19] In fact, the FFMC was so concerned about this issue that the FFMC Code of Practice specifically states that decisions about the method and timing of the abortion must not be influenced by the possibility of foetal tissue use, nor should the possibility of foetal tissue use alter the treatment of a woman who has a spontaneous abortion, or whose foetus dies *in utero*.[20] This is important since there is evidence that the suitability of tissues for certain procedures is affected by the particular method of abortion used.[21]

Targeting is even more of a problem given the FFMC's view of moral status. To give a hypothetical example, suppose that a pregnant woman finds out that her existing child, who is terminally ill, could be saved by the use of foetal tissue. She

[17] *Ibid.*
[18] See Cannold, *The Abortion Myth*, pp. 7–8.
[19] Another way to view the separation of the abortion decision from any subsequent decision about the use of foetal tissue is to see it as a standard response to a conflict of interest. A discussion of some of the conflict of interest problems that arise in medicine can be found in Stephen R. Latham, 'Conflict of Interest in Medical Practice', in Michael Davis and Andrew Stark (eds), *Conflict of Interest in the Professions*, (New York: Oxford, 2001).
[20] Code of Practice paragraph 3.2, in Polkinghorne, 'Law and Ethics of Transplanting Foetal Tissue', p. 332.
[21] See, for example, McCullagh, *The Foetus as Transplant Donor*, pp. 105–108.

might well be so concerned about the existing child, and so desperate for them to receive this treatment, that she demands that her foetus be terminated and the tissues used to save her existing child. Since the welfare of existing children can be taken into account when determining the legality of abortion in the United Kingdom, the mere existence of the treatment and the possibility of targeting would have not only induced this woman to abort, but also made the abortion legal. Anyone who holds that the rights of the foetus are in any way similar to those of a child or adult would be concerned about this possibility.

The FFMC was also concerned about the possibility of creating a child using the ovarian tissue of a dead foetus. They felt that this was ethically problematic, and effectively banned this type of research by insisting upon an intermediary between the source and user of foetal tissues. The FFMC believed that specific consent from the mother of the foetus would be necessary before anyone could create a child used the foetus' ovarian tissue; as specific consent is impossible through an intermediary (in this particular case the tissue bank established as a result of the FFMC's recommendations) the possibility of using foetal ovarian tissue to initiate a pregnancy is effectively ruled out.[22] However, why they felt that this issue was so intensely problematic is never explained, though I assume that they were worried about the effect it might have on such children later in life to learn that their genetic mother was an aborted foetus.

The FFMC's insistence that consent must be obtained from the mother for the use of any foetal materials was also not uncontroversial, given that some people believe that the decision to abort severs any bond of responsibility between the mother and the foetus.[23] The FFMC were of the view that this is too dismissive of the complexities of the abortion decision:

> Because abortion is a decision of moral ambiguity and perplexity for many, reached only through a conflict of considerations, it seems too harsh a judgement of the mother's relation to her foetus to suppose that she is no longer in a special position with regard to it, following an abortion.[24]

It is also undeniably true that the use of foetal material may lead to certain discoveries of immense importance for the mother. For example, if the foetus was found to be HIV positive, or suffering from hepatitis, then it follows that the mother must also be suffering from these same conditions, even if she is unaware of it. Such issues make it reasonable to insist that the mother's informed consent be obtained before any foetal tissues are used in research or treatments.

---

[22] See Polkinghorne, 'Law and Ethics of Transplanting Foetal Tissue', p. 328.
[23] *Ibid.*
[24] FFMC Report, paragraph 2.8, quoted in Polkinghorne, 'Law and Ethics of Transplanting Foetal Tissue', p. 328.

Problems with the FFMC Report

Having discussed briefly the main concerns of the FFMC, I will now turn my attention to the problems with the report, the most obvious problem being the FFMC's definition of moral status. As I have already mentioned, the FFMC decided that it was not necessary to answer questions such as whether the foetus is a person, or other questions usually considered when attempting to determine foetal status, but instead they asked (and answered) the different question 'How is it right to treat the human embryo (and foetus)?'[25] The FFMC decided that 'On the basis of its potential to develop into a human being, a foetus is entitled to respect, according it a status broadly comparable to that of a living person'.[26] The problem with asking such a question, and with asserting the answer that they did, is that the question cannot be answered without first determining foetal status, and that the answer that they gave to the question *assumes* a particular view of foetal status. The view of foetal status that they have implicitly assumed is that potential personhood grants a being all, or nearly all, of the rights of personhood, and that abortion is synonymous with foetal evacuation, not foetal death. Obviously this is a view with which I disagree.

To illustrate the problem of trying to answer the question 'How is it right to treat the human embryo?' without first examining its moral status, consider the difficulties of answering the question 'How is it right to treat kakapo?' without knowing what kakapo is. It could be a mineral, in which case talking about how to treat it seems rather pointless. It could be an animal, in which case knowing what it is like will make a great deal of difference to how it is decided to treat it: consider the difference in the way that cockroaches and dogs are treated. It could be a disease, in which case the question takes on a whole new meaning, for in talking about how to treat kakapo the question becomes one of how to restore to good health a person who is afflicted with kakapo. It could be a parasite, a plant, a new type of car, or an alien life form. In order to appropriately answer the question of how to treat it, it is vital to be clear about what is being discussed.

In fact, the kakapo is an extremely endangered flightless parrot, now only found on a couple of small isolated islands near the South Island of New Zealand. As of 1990, there were about 40 kakapos left in the world, all of them living in protected habitats on these small islands, having been relocated from larger islands by the New Zealand Department of Conservation in order to prevent the extinction of the species.[27] Knowing this about the kakapo makes it possible to answer the question of how to treat kakapo. Without knowing this, the question is impossible

---

[25] From the report of the Warnock Committee, paragraph 11.9, quoted in Polkinghorne, 'Law and Ethics of Transplanting Foetal Tissue', *ibid*, p. 325, my insert.

[26] FFMC report paragraph 9.1, quoted in Polkinghorne, 'Law and Ethics of Transplanting Foetal Tissue', *ibid.*

[27] For a description of the kakapo and the attempts to prevent its extinction, see Douglas Adams and Mark Carwardine, *Last Chance to See* ..., (London: Heinemann, 1990), pp. 99–135.

to answer. In a similar way, it is obviously futile to attempt to answer the question of how we ought to treat the human embryo and foetus without knowing a great deal about it. Questions of its moral status need to be examined, and whether it is a person or not, or whether it has the potential to become a person, will be essential parts of this examination.

Thus I would disagree with the FFMC's answer to the question, as I believe they have relied on inaccurate assumptions about foetal status. In addition, their view of the moral status of the embryo and foetus seems to entail that the moral status of the embryo is the same as that of the foetus, and that this value does not change during pregnancy. This is clearly illustrated by Polkinghorne's suggestion that it is not ethically acceptable to create embryos solely for the purpose of research, because this means that the embryo is not being treated in a manner broadly comparable to children and adults.[28] As I have already argued, while the embryo does have the potential to become a person, this potential is a long way from being realised, and thus I would argue that the moral status of the embryo is much less than the moral status of a near-term foetus.

While the FFMC used a poor argument in reaching its decision, I agree with the decision that they made. In this particular case, they reached the right conclusion, but by the wrong argument. I will therefore consider what arguments might be used to justify the position taken by the FFMC, and if these arguments also apply to the use of partial ectogenesis for the purpose of creating organs for transplant surgery.

A Better Argument for Restrictions on Foetal Tissue Use

The two main restrictions the FFMC placed on the use of foetal tissue were, (1), that the decision to abort be kept separate from the decision to allow foetal tissue use, and, (2), that the consent of the mother was necessary before foetal tissues could be used for any purpose.

Of these two conditions, I think it is the first one that is most open to argument. An argument in favour of the second restriction, that the mother's consent is required before any tissues are used, is easily supplied. The argument that use of foetal tissues does *not* require the mother's consent is based upon the idea that the mother is abrogating any responsibility for the foetus through the act of abortion. I have argued at length that this is precisely *not* what is happening, but rather that what happens in an abortion is that a woman *does* take responsibility for the life of the foetus, and decides that this particular could-be child is better off not being born into these circumstances at this particular time. Based on this position, it is obvious that the consent of the mother would be required before any foetal tissues are utilised for research or treatment purposes.

Thus if the requirement for a woman's consent can be justified, we are left only with the first requirement of the FFMC, that the decision to abort and the decision

---

[28] Polkinghorne, 'Law and Ethics of Transplanting Foetal Tissue', p. 326.

to allow usage of foetal tissues be kept as separate as possible, even at the cost of making the foetal tissues unusable (as would be the case if the method of abortion was incompatible with the particular research to be undertaken). What reasons might there be for thinking that it is appropriate to keep separate the decision to abort and the decision to allow the use of foetal tissues, apart from reasons based on a faulty view of the moral status of the foetus? I suggest that the most important factor that must be taken into consideration here is the means by which abortion is justified in the first place.

If abortion can only be justified by appeal to the woman's right to bodily autonomy, then this does not entail a right to secure the death of the foetus. In this sort of situation, it is not only reasonable, but obligatory, to ensure that abortion is only undertaken for the benefit of the mother. Thus it is also ethically required to ensure that there is no possibility of pressure being applied to the mother to abort for reasons other than for her own well-being. This leads naturally to an insistence on separation between decisions to abort and decisions regarding the subsequent use of foetal tissues. This is, of course, the exact position taken by the FFMC. But what about the possibility of some other basis for a right to an abortion? I have argued at some length that the parents of some could-be child have a right to demand its death during an abortion, on the grounds of either a right not to be a parent (in the general case) or for the benefit of the could-be child itself (in cases where abortion is sought for foetal deformity). What are the implications of this view for subsequent use of foetal tissue? Is there a need in these cases to insist on the separation of the abortion decision and a decision about later use of foetal tissue? I argue that in these cases too it would be unethical to allow the possibility of later use of foetal tissue to affect the decision whether or not to abort. Let us consider first the right not to be a parent, and its implications for use of foetal tissue.

Foetal Tissue Use and the Right to Not be a Parent

In examining the right not to be a parent, I concluded that this right did exist as an aspect of personal autonomy. I also suggested that it allowed a parent to demand the death of the foetus under certain circumstances, since being forced to become a parent against one's will is a violation of autonomy. I also suggested that the reason that the parents, and only the parents, had the right to demand the death of the foetus is because of the special relationship that they will have, or will be expected to have, with this developing human after birth. When examining the right not to become a parent in this way, it can be seen that this right is actually connected to the future benefit of the child. Consider the following quote from Steven Ross, which I discussed earlier:

> A woman may feel very strongly that she and not anyone else ought to raise whatever children she brings into the world. Or, more likely, that she ought to do so only in

conjunction with a supportive husband who is also (and not by chance) the father of the child.[29]

What Ross is essentially suggesting is that a person who is asserting their right not to become a parent, by demanding the death of the foetus, is doing so partly for the benefit of that child. The circumstances in which the person finds themself are not ideal for raising the child, and so they assert their right not to become a parent *because* they do not want their child to be raised in those circumstances.

It is also extremely important that the right not to become a parent is part of the right to autonomy. Being forced to become a parent against your will is a violation of autonomy, but being pressured to abort to provide a benefit to someone else is *also* a violation of autonomy.

These considerations give us two reasons for thinking that the decision to abort should be kept separate from any decision about subsequent use of foetal tissues. First, since the decision to abort is made partly for the benefit of the could-be child, it is their benefit, not someone else's, that should be considered in a decision as to whether or not to end their life. Second, since the right to not become a parent is an aspect of autonomy, it should be protected from any pressures, since these pressures are in themselves a violation of that autonomy.

Foetal Tissue Use and Abortions for Foetal Defect

The second case that I mentioned where the parents may demand the death of the foetus is in the case of foetal defect or deformity. As I argued earlier when discussing abortion,[30] decisions to abort in such cases are decisions made for the benefit of the future child. The parents have made the decision that the life of the could-be child is not worth starting, and thus they decide to prevent a future child from coming into existence by securing its death through abortion. Should the decision to abort be separate from any decision to use foetal tissues in these sorts of cases? A decision to abort due to foetal defect is a decision made for the benefit of the future child, with some carry-over benefits for the parents, who would have to care for the disabled child. It is not, and should not, be a decision made to benefit a third party. A decision that the life of this future child is not worth starting should be reached without thought of possible benefits to any third parties.[31]

[29] *Ibid.*, p. 240.
[30] See 'Abortion Due to Foetal Defect', in the previous chapter.
[31] Note that this only rules out creating a foetus with the intention of abortion; it does not rule out creating a child who would be capable of providing some necessary blood or tissue donations after birth. Thus my arguments here would not apply to parents who conceived a child in the hope of producing (for example) a child that would be a compatible bone marrow donor for an existing sibling who required such a transplant.

Therefore I would agree with the restrictions placed on the use of foetal tissue by the FFMC while disagreeing with the reasons that they gave for those restrictions.

Decisions about abortions should be kept separate from decisions about the later use of foetal tissues, since in all cases the abortion decision should only be concerned with the welfare of the future could-be child and the parents of that child, and not with the welfare of other parties who may benefit from the abortion. Pressures on women to abort are a violation of the autonomy of the pregnant woman in any case, and so steps should be taken to minimise the risk of such pressure occurring. I also argued that the consent of the mother is required for the use of any foetal tissue, for the decision to abort is not a decision to abrogate responsibility for the foetus, but rather to accept moral responsibility through abortion. The FFMC's recommendation that an intermediary control the use of foetal tissues in these cases is a necessary safeguard on the autonomy of those who must make decisions about the use of those foetal tissues.

Having argued for these conditions in the case of foetal tissue obtained after an abortion, I now intend to apply those arguments to the issue at hand, the use of partial ectogenesis for the purpose of providing organs for transplant.

Partial Ectogenesis for Transplant Revisited

As I mentioned earlier, for anyone to even consider partial ectogenesis for transplant as an option, it is necessary to base that decision on a theory that allows abortion on some grounds other than merely preserving the bodily autonomy of the mother, since partial ectogenesis for transplant entails the death of the foetus without the existence of a gestational mother whose rights must be protected. While I have argued that there are other arguments that justify seeking the death of the foetus in an abortion, I would suggest that none of these arguments would be sufficient to allow the use of partial ectogenesis for transplant.

In discussing the FFMC's restrictions on the use of foetal tissues, I have argued that only after a decision that it is morally appropriate to end the life of the foetus should there be any consideration of whether tissues from that foetus should be used in research or treatment. It would be quite impossible to justify partial ectogenesis for transplant on these grounds, for the life of the foetus in these situations would not be ended were it not for the fact that it could be used to provide organs for transplant surgery. In partial ectogenesis for transplant, the decision to end the life of the foetus and the decision to use its tissues for transplant purposes can *never* be kept separate, since the life of the foetus is ended for no reason other than the need for transplantable organs.

Foetal Status and Partial Ectogenesis

However, using partial ectogenesis for transplant purposes might possibly be justified in one other way. In discussing the status of the embryo and foetus, I suggested that the foetus gains in moral standing as it develops, but that early on in pregnancy, it has little intrinsic moral standing. If this is the case, then perhaps partial ectogenesis for transplant might be justified on this basis. Since in this case there is never any intention of there being social parents whose interests must be protected, the death of the foetus could be justified merely on the grounds that it lacks significant moral standing. I have argued that the *in utero* foetus gains a good deal of moral standing from the relationship it bears to its parents, particularly its mother, thus in cases where there is no relationship the foetus does not have significant moral standing to prevent it being killed for the benefit of others.

Unfortunately for the proponents of partial ectogenesis for transplant, I do not think that this argument will succeed. If the foetus has developed to a point where the organs have differentiated sufficiently to be useful for the purposes of transplant, even if this only means that they can be removed to be placed in a special environment to grow to adult size, then I would suggest that the moral status of the foetus is sufficient to prevent its death in all cases where it is not otherwise justified by the foetus' own interests.

I argued in an earlier chapter that the potential of the developing embryo and foetus is of particular importance, and that this importance increases during the course of pregnancy. I also suggested that there are some crucial obstacles on the path to realisation of potential, and successful negotiation of each of these would seem to increase the moral status of the resulting developing human. The examples that I gave were fertilisation and implantation. Both of these are crucial steps in the development of the embryo, and both dramatically increase the chances of realisation of the potential for personhood. For a foetus to develop to the stage where its organs are of use, it must have passed through both of these vital stages, and if left to its own devices, the foetus will have a high probability of realising its potential. Thus I would suggest that any foetus that is suitable to become an organ donor has already reached a stage of development where its moral status is sufficient to prevent its being killed, except in special, and limited, circumstances; circumstances that will always be in some way aimed at the benefit of the foetus itself. However, if the potential for personhood were to be permanently removed, such as by inducing severe brain damage, then this might allow a way around the argument that I have just outlined. In that case it may be necessary to rely on consequentialist arguments, such as the one proposed by Singer and Wells, if one wanted to argue against the use of partial ectogenesis for transplant.

There is one final argument against the idea of using partial ectogenesis for transplant that comes, indirectly, from Steven Ross. I suggested a moment ago that in cases where there is no relationship with potential social parents to worry about, that the foetus does not have significant enough moral standing to prevent it being killed for the benefit of others. However, as Ross pointed out, the special relationship that a foetus has with its potential parents cuts both ways.

It is rarely noticed that only the parent's desire to see the foetus dead is ever taken seriously in the first place; no one else could possibly have a reason we would consider for a moment.[32]

The special relationship that the foetus has with its parents gives it extra moral status that makes its killing a serious matter. But it is the possibility of that relationship that also gives the only realistic justification for killing the foetus. If anyone other than the parents was to insist that the foetus be killed, it would not even be considered. In the absence of anyone who will fulfil that parental role, there does not seem to be anyone who can possibly justify killing the foetus.

In Summary

While the idea of being able to provide virtually unlimited organs for transplant through partial ectogenesis might seem to be attractive, I do not think that the procedure can be justified. There are many arguments against it, any one of which is probably significant enough to prevent the procedure. There is some evidence that most people would have a preference that foetuses should not be created and used in this way, which should be sufficient reason for preference utilitarians to abandon the idea. In addition, none of the usual justifications for killing a foetus seem to apply in this case. The right for a person not to become a parent does not apply, nor does killing the foetus for its own benefit. In any case, a foetus that is sufficiently developed to be a candidate for organ donation of any sort would seem to have sufficient moral status to prevent anyone killing it in the absence of the pressing rights of others.

---

[32] 'Abortion and the Death of the Foetus', p. 244.

Chapter 9

Conclusions

The development of ectogenesis would have implications in a number of areas. Development of this technology would bring the greatest change to infertility treatment since the advent of medicine, it could conceivably lead to severe restrictions on a woman's right to an abortion, and it could lead to enormous numbers of embryos being created solely for the purpose of providing organs for transplant. What conclusions can we draw about the ethical implications of this technology, and how should we deal with it, if and when it is developed?

As far as using ectogenesis as an infertility treatment goes, I can see no objection to the use of ectogenesis, though there does seem to be a strong objection with regard to the funding of the research to develop ectogenesis. As I argued in Chapter 4, the suggestion that ectogenesis is unnatural, and the suggestion that its development would bring us closer to *Brave New World* both seem to be unfounded. Provided that children gestated in the device develop normally, which is a purely empirical question that needs to be answered, then there also is no valid objection to the use of the device based on the harm that would come to the future child through being conceived and gestated in this way.

As far as objections to the development (as opposed to the use) of ectogenesis goes, I have argued that the suggestion that adoption should be preferred to ectogenesis is unfounded, and that feminist concerns about the development of such technologies would be best addressed by women being fully involved in the development and use of these technologies. There does seem to be a strong argument against the use of public monies in the development of ectogenesis, for this type of research does seem to be a low priority as far as medical research goes. As long as the health budget is limited, then ectogenetic research would be of direct benefit to few enough people that it would be unlikely to receive public funding. However, I can see no direct objection to the use of private funds to stimulate research in this area.

If an ectogenetic device was developed that was able to take over the gestation of an existing foetus, then this would have enormous implications for the care and treatment of newborns, for ante-natal care, and in the area of abortion ethics. I have argued that the existence of such a device would be of benefit to some women, who desire to parent, but who may be forced to abort for maternal health reasons. These are cases where the desire for an abortion is a desire to end the pregnancy, rather than to end the life of the foetus.

However, in most abortion cases, the aim is not simply to end the pregnancy, but rather to ensure that there will be no future child. While some might argue that in such cases we have a duty to preserve the life of the foetus if this is possible, I have argued that this is not the case. The right to an abortion is more than simply a right to bodily integrity, and the morality of abortion decisions cannot be determined without a detailed examination of foetal moral status. I have argued at length in Chapter 6 for a moderate view of foetal status (that the foetus has little intrinsic status at conception, but that its moral value grows during pregnancy), coupled with a recognition of the significance of the relationship between a foetus and its parents. This grants a woman the right to demand the death of the foetus that she is carrying, on the grounds of her right not to be a parent. While an ectogenetic device could preserve the life of the foetus in such cases, the foetus' lack of significant intrinsic moral status means that the wishes of the parents should be fulfilled.

In cases where there is no person who can realistically be said to be the future parent of a foetus, then I have suggested that the intrinsic moral status of the foetus is sufficient to prevent its being killed. This effectively rules out the possibility of using ectogenetic technology to gestate embryos solely for the purpose of producing donor organs for transplant surgery. While the greatest part of the moral status of the foetus comes by virtue of the potential for future relationship with its parents, its intrinsic moral status is sufficient to prevent anyone other than its parents from seeking its death.

How Should we Deal with Ectogenesis?

When ectogenesis is being used as an infertility treatment, I would suggest that it could be treated as being simply another form of reproductive technology. Regulations that apply to other forms of reproductive technology could be easily adapted to apply to ectogenesis. When being utilised in this way, ectogenesis raises few new ethical issues.

However, the fact that the development of ectogenesis could lead to restrictions on a woman's right to an abortion is an alarming possibility. Having argued that abortion is properly seen as ensuring that there will be no future child, rather than merely ensuring the integrity of one's bodily boundaries, I would like to see the right to not become a parent given some form of legal protection. This would then allow parents to secure the death of the foetus in an abortion, at least in the earlier stages of foetal development.

The possibility that ectogenetic technology could be used as a means of creating organs for transplant is also disturbing. However, all that is necessary to prevent this from happening is some simple legislation that guarantees clear separation between the death of a donor and any subsequent use of their organs and tissues.[1] Such legislation would prevent anyone from creating embryos for the purpose of procuring organs for the purpose of transplant.

While ectogenesis raises many ethical issues, few of these issues are really new. The main benefit of examining the ethical implications of its development is

---

[1] Such as the United Kingdom's FFMC Code of Practice. See Chapter 8.

the fact that it focuses our attention on those aspects of the issue that are really of central importance, most notably the status of the embryo and foetus. Once the issue of the moral status of the embryo and foetus is resolved, the actual ethical implications of ectogenesis are clearly revealed.

Bibliography

Adams, Douglas and Carwardine, Mark, *Last Chance to See* ..., (London: Heinemann, 1990).

Almond, Brenda, 'Rights' in Peter Singer, (ed.), *A Companion to Ethics*, (Oxford: Basil Blackwell, 1993).

Bankowski, Zbigniew, 'International Ethical Guidelines for Biomedical Research Involving Human Subjects', in *Ethics and Research on Human Subjects: International Guidelines*, Geneva: CIOMS, 1993.

Bartlett, R.H. and Gazzaniga, A.B., 'Extracorporeal Circulation for Cardiopulmonary Failure', *Current Problems in Surgery*, 15 (1978), pp. 1–96.

Bartlett, Robert et al., 'Extracorporeal Circulation in Neonatal Respiratory Failure: A Prospective Randomised Study', *Pediatrics*, 76 (1985), pp. 479–87.

_____, 'Extracorporeal Membrane Oxygenation for Newborn Respiratory Failure: Forty-five Cases', *Surgery*, 92 (1982), pp. 425–33.

Bayles, Michael, *Reproductive Ethics*, (Englewood Cliffs: Prentice–Hall, 1984).

Bayne, Tim, 'Abortion and the Immorality of Killing: How Far Back do I Go?', presented at the International Conference on Applied Ethics, Hong Kong, December 1999.

Benatar, David, 'The Wrong of Wrongful Life', *American Philosophical Quarterly*, 37 (2000), pp. 175–83 .

_____, 'Why it is Better Never to Come into Existence', *American Philosophical Quarterly*, 34 (1997), pp. 345–55.

Bigelow, John and Pargetter, Robert, 'Morality, Potential Persons and Abortion', *American Philosophical Quarterly*, 25 (1988), pp. 173–81.

Blandau, Richard, 'In Vitro Fertilisation and Embryo Transfer', *Fertility and Infertility*, 33 (1980), pp. 3–111.

Buckle, Stephen, 'Arguing from Potential', in Singer et al. (eds), *Embryo Experimentation*, (Melbourne: Cambridge University, 1990).

Bulletti, Carlo et al., 'Early Human Pregnancy in vitro Utilising an Artificially Perfused Uterus', *Fertility and Sterility*, 49 (1988), pp. 991–6.

Callaghan, John and Angeles, Jose Delos, 'Long Term Extracorporeal Circulation in the Development of an Artificial Placenta for Respiratory Distress of the Newborn', *Surgical Forum*, 12 (1961), pp. 215–17.

Callaghan, John et al., 'Studies on Lambs of the Development of an Artificial Placenta: Review of Nine Long–Term Survivors of Extracorporeal Circulation Maintained in a Fluid Medium', *Canadian Journal of Surgery*, 8 (1965), pp. 208–13.

_____, 'Study of Prepulmonary Bypass in the Development of an Artificial Placenta for Prematurity and Respiratory Distress Syndrome of the Newborn', *Journal of Thoracic and Cardiovascular Surgery*, 44 (1962), pp. 600–607.

Callahan, Daniel, *New York Times*, 27 July 1978, p. A16.

Callahan, Joan C., 'Ensuring a Stillborn: The Ethics of Lethal Injection in Late Abortion', in Joan C. Callahan (ed.), *Reproduction, Ethics, and the Law: Feminist Perspectives*, (Bloomington: Indiana University, 1995).

Cannold, Leslie, *The Abortion Myth: Feminism, Morality and the Hard Choices Women Make*, (St Leonards: Allen and Unwin, 1998).

_____, 'Women, Ectogenesis and Ethical Theory', *Journal of Applied Philosophy*, 12 (1995), pp. 55–64.

_____, *Women's Response to Ectogenesis, and the Relevance of Severance Abortion Theory*, (Masters Thesis: Monash University, 1992).

Chamberlain, Geoffrey, 'An Artificial Placenta: The Development of an Extracorporeal System for Maintenance of Immature Infants with Respiratory Problems', *American Journal of Obstetrics and Gynaecology*, 100 (1968), pp. 615–26.

Chartrand, Sabra, 'Patents', *New York Times*, 19 July 1993, p. D2.

Chemke, Juan and Steinberg, Avraham, 'Ethics and Medical Genetic in Israel', in Dorothy C. Wertz and John C. Fletcher (eds), *Ethics and Human Genetics: A Cross–Cultural Perspective*, (Berlin: Springer-Verlag, 1989), pp. 271–84.

Christman, John, 'Introduction', in John Christman (ed.), *The Inner Citadel*, (Oxford: Oxford University, 1989).

Coleman, Stephen, 'Thought Experiments and Personal Identity', *Philosophical Studies*, 98 (2000), pp. 53–69.

_____, 'A Surrogate for Surrogacy? – The Artificial Uterus', *Australian Journal of Professional and Applied Ethics*, 1 (1999), pp. 49–60.

_____, 'Would You Like a Coffee? Slippery Slopes, Gratuities and Corruption in Police Work', *Professional Ethics*, 6 (1998), pp. 107–22.

Cooper, William, 'Placental Chamber – Artificial Uterus', United States Patent number 5,218,958, filed 21 February 1991; granted 15 June, 1993; column 1.

Corea, Gena, *The Mother Machine*, (London: The Women's Press, 1985/1988).

Cubbon, John, 'The Principle of QALY Maximisation as the Basis for Allocating Health Care Resources', *Journal of Medical Ethics*, 17 (1991), pp. 181–4.

Daniels, Cynthia R., *At Women's Expense: State Power and the Politics of Foetal Rights*, (Cambridge MA: Harvard University, 1993).

Davis, Nancy Ann, 'Contemporary Deontology' in Peter Singer (ed.), *A Companion to Ethics*, (Oxford: Basil Blackwell, 1993).

Davis v Davis v King E–14496 (Fifth Ct. Tennessee), Young, Judge (1989).

Dawson, Karen, 'Fertilisation and Moral Status: A Scientific Perspective', in *Embryo Experimentation*, Singer et al. (eds), (Cambridge UK: Cambridge University, 1990).

_____, 'Introduction: An Outline of Scientific Aspects of Human Embryo Research', in *Embryo Experimentation*, Singer et al. (eds), (Cambridge UK: Cambridge University, 1990).

_____, 'Segmentation and Moral Status: A Scientific Perspective', in *Embryo Experimentation*, Singer et al. (eds), (Cambridge UK: Cambridge University, 1990).

DeKretser, David et al., 'Transfer of a Human Zygote', *The Lancet*, 2 (1973), pp. 728–9.

Deykin, Eva Y. et al., 'The Postadoption Experience of Surrendering Parents', *American Journal of Orthopsychiatry*, 54 (1984), p. 273.

Donohue, John and Levitt, Steven, 'Legalised Abortion and Crime', (1999), unpublished manuscript, available from the authors at Stanford University, and the University of Chicago.

Dworkin, Ronald, *Life's Dominion*, (London: HarperCollins, 1995).

Edwards, Robert, *A Matter of Life*, (London: Sphere, 1981).

Firestone, Shulamith, *The Dialectic of Sex*, (New York: Bantam, 1971).

Fitzgerald, Laurence, 'Test Tube Morality in the Final Analysis', *The Advocate*, (Melbourne) 5 April, 1982.

Freitas, Robert A. Jr, 'Foetal Adoption: A Technological Solution to the Problem of Abortion Ethics', *The Humanist*, May/June 1980, pp. 22–3.

Fried, Charles, *Right and Wrong*, (Cambridge MA: Harvard University, 1978).

Glover, Jonathon, *Causing Death and Saving Lives*, (Harmondsworth: Penguin, 1977).

Goodin, Robert E., 'Utility and the Good', in Peter Singer, (ed.), *A Companion to Ethics*, (Oxford: Basil Blackwell, 1993).

Griffith, Bartley P. et al, 'Arteriovenous ECMO for Neonatal Respiratory Support: A Study in Perigestational Lambs', *The Journal of Thoracic and Cardiovascular Surgery*, 77 (1979), pp. 595–601.

Groeber, Walter R., 'Antiabruption Dynamics of the Intervillous Circulation in an Artificial Uterus', *American Journal of Obstetrics* and Gynaecology, 95 (1966), pp. 640–647.

Hadfield, Peter, 'Japanese Pioneers Raise Kid in Rubber Womb', *New Scientist*, (25 April 1992), p. 5.

Harris, John, 'Unprincipled QALYs: A Response to Cubbon', *Journal of Medical Ethics*, 17 (1991), pp. 185–8.

Herbenick, Raymond, 'Remarks on Abortion, Abandonment and Adoption Opportunities', *Philosophy and Public Affairs*, 5 (1975), pp. 98–104.

Hursthouse, Rosalind, *Beginning Lives*, (Oxford: Basil Blackwell, 1987).

Huxley, Aldous, *Brave New World*, (London: Chatto and Windus, 1932), reprinted modern edition (London: Flamingo Modern Classics, 1994).

James, David N., 'Artificial Insemination: A Re-Examination', *Philosophy and Theology*, 2 (1988), pp. 305–26.

_____, 'Ectogenesis: A Reply to Singer and Wells', *Bioethics*, 1 (1987), pp. 80–99.

Jamieson, Dale, 'When Utilitarians Should Be Virtue Theorists: The Case of Global Environmental Change', presented at the International Conference on Applied Ethics, Hong Kong, December 1999.

Jersild, Paul J., 'On Having Children: A Theological and Moral Analysis of *In Vitro* Fertilisation', in Edward D. Schneider, (ed.), *Questions About the Beginning of Life*, (Minneapolis: Augsburg, 1985).

Kamm, Frances, *Creation and Abortion: A Study in Moral and Legal Philosophy*, (New York: Oxford, 1992).

Kant, Immanuel, *Foundations of the Metaphysics of Morals*, trans. L. W. Beck, (New York, Macmillan, 1990).

Kass, Leon, 'The New Biology: What Price Relieving Man's Estate?', *Journal of the American Medical Association*, 174 (19 November 1971), pp. 779–88.

_____, 'Babies by Means of In Vitro Fertilisation: Unethical Experiments on the Unborn?', *New England Journal of Medicine*, 285 (1971), pp. 1174–9.

Krantz, Kermit et al., 'Physiology of Maternal-Foetal Relationship Through the Extracorporeal Circulation of the Human Placenta', *American Journal of Obstetrics and Gynaecology*, 83 (1962), pp. 1214–28.

Kuwabara, Yoshinori et al., 'Development of an Artificial Placenta: Survival of Isolated Goat Foetuses for Three Weeks with Umbilical Arteriovenous Extracorporeal Membrane Oxygenation', *Artificial Organs*, 17 (1993), pp. 996–1003.

_____, 'Artificial Placenta: Long-Term Extrauterine Incubation of Isolated Goat Foetuses', *Artificial Organs*, 13 (1989), pp. 527–31.

_____, 'Development of Extrauterine Foetal Incubation System Using Extracorporeal Membrane Oxygenator', *Artificial Organs*, 11 (1987), pp. 224–7.

Lauritzen, Paul, *Pursuing Parenthood*, (Bloomington: Indiana University, 1993).

Mackenzie, Catriona, 'Abortion and Embodiment', *Australian Journal of Philosophy*, 70 (1992), pp. 136–55.

Mahoney, Joan, 'Adoption as a Feminist Alternative to Reproductive Technology', in Joan
        C. Callahan (ed.), *Reproduction, Ethics and the Law*, (Bloomington: Indiana
        University, 1995).
Marlow, John, *US News and World Report*, 7 August 1978, p. 24.
Marquis, Don, 'Justifying the Rights of Pregnancy: The Interest View', *Criminal Justice
        Ethics*, 13 (1994), pp. 67–81.
_____, 'Why Abortion is Immoral', *Journal of Philosophy*, 76 (1989), pp. 183–202.
McCullagh, Peter, *The Foetus as Transplant Donor: Scientific, Social and Ethical
        Perspectives*, (Chichester: John Wiley and Sons, 1987).
McInerney, Peter, 'Does a Foetus Already Have a Future-Like-Ours?', *Journal of
        Philosophy*, 87 (1990), pp. 264–8.
Morreall, John, 'Of Marsupials and Men: A Thought Experiment on Abortion', *Dialogos*, 37
        (1981), pp. 7–18.
Murata, Yuji et al., 'Cardiac Oxygenation by Extracorporeal Membrane Oxygenation in
        Exteriorised Foetal Lambs', *American Journal of Obstetrics* and *Gynaecology*,
        174 (1996), pp. 864–70.
Murphy, Julien S., 'Is Pregnancy Necessary? Feminist Concerns about Ectogenesis',
        Hypatia, 3 (1989), pp. 65–84.
NHMRC, 'Services for the Termination of Pregnancy in Australia: A Review', *Draft
        Consultation Document, September 1995.*
Nelson, Hilde Lindemann and Nelson, James Lindemann, 'Cutting Motherhood in Two:
        Some Suspicions Concerning Surrogacy', in Helen Bequaert Holmes and Laura
        M. Purdy (eds), *Feminist Perspectives in Medical Ethics*, (Bloomington: Indiana
        University, 1992).
Norcross, Alastair, 'Killing, Abortion, and Contraception: A Reply to Marquis', *Journal of
        Philosophy*, 87 (1990), pp. 268–77.
Oakley, Justin, 'Varieties of Virtue Ethics', *Ratio*, 9 (1996), pp. 128–52.
O'Neill, Onora, 'Kantian Ethics', in Peter Singer (ed.), *A Companion to Ethics*, (Oxford:
        Basil Blackwell, 1993).
Overall, Christine, *Ethics and Human Reproduction: A Feminist Analysis*, (Boston: Allen
        and Unwin, 1987).
_____, 'Frozen Embryos and "Father's Rights": Parenthood and Decision-Making in the
        Cryopreservation of Embryos', in Joan C. Callahan (ed.), *Reproduction, Ethics,
        and the Law: Feminist Perspectives*, (Bloomington: Indiana University, 1995).
Parfit, Derek, *Reasons and Persons*, (Oxford: Oxford University, 1984).
Paske, Gerald H., 'Sperm-Napping and the Right Not to Have a Child', *Australasian
        Journal of Philosophy*, 65 (1987), pp. 98–103.
Pence, Gregory, *Classic Cases in Medical Ethics*, 2nd ed., (New York: McGraw–Hill,
        1995).
_____, 'Virtue Theory', in Peter Singer (ed.), *A Companion to Ethics*, (Oxford: Basil
        Blackwell, 1993).
Pettit, Philip, 'Consequentialism', in Peter Singer (ed.), *A Companion to Ethics*, (Oxford:
        Basil Blackwell, 1993).
Polkinghorne, J. C., 'Law and Ethics of Transplanting Foetal Tissue', in Robert G. Edwards
        (ed.), *Foetal Tissue Transplants in Medicine*, (Cambridge: Cambridge University,
        1992).
Purdy, Laura, 'The Morality of New Reproductive Technologies', in *Reproducing Persons*,
        (Ithaca: Cornell University, 1996).
Rachels, James, 'Active and Passive Euthanasia', in James Rachels (ed.), *Moral Problems*
        3rd Ed., (New York: Harper and Row, 1979).

Ramsey, Paul, 'Reference Points in Deciding About Abortion', in J.T. Noonan (ed.), *The Morality of Abortion*, (Harvard University: Cambridge MA, 1970).

Raymond, Janice, 'Of Ice and Men: The Big Chill over Women's Reproductive Rights', *Issues in Reproductive and Genetic Engineering: Journal of International Feminist Analysis*, 3 (1990), p. 49.

Rivkin, Jeremy and Howard, Ted, *Who Shall Play God?*, (New York: Dell, 1977).

Robertson, John, *Children of Choice*, (Princeton: Princeton University, 1994).

Ross, Steven, 'Abortion and the Death of the Foetus', *Philosophy and Public Affairs*, 11 (1982), pp. 232–45.

Rothman, Barbara Katz, *Recreating Motherhood: Ideology and Technology in a Patriarchal Society*, (New York: N.W. Norton, 1989).

Rowland, Robyn, *Living Laboratories*, (Sydney: Pan, 1992).

_____, 'Motherhood, Patriarchal Power, Alienation and the Issue of "Choice" in Sex Preselection', in Patricia Spallone and Deborah Lynn Steinberg (eds), *Made to Order: The Myth of Reproductive and Genetic Progress*, (Oxford: Pergamon, 1987).

Sarin, C.L. et al., 'Further Development of an Artificial Placenta with the use of Membrane Oxygenator and Venovenous Perfusion', *Surgery*, 60 (1966), pp. 754–60.

SenGupta, A., et al, 'An Artificial Placenta Designed to Maintain Life During Cardiorespiratory Distress', *Transactions: American Society for Artificial Internal Organs*, 10 (1964), pp. 63–5.

Sheehan, Maureen and Wells, Deane, 'The Allocation of Medical Resources', in *Medical Care and Markets*, C.L. Buchanan and E.W. Prior (eds), (Sydney: Allen and Unwin, 1985).

Shickle, Darren, 'Public Preferences for Health Care: Prioritisation in the United Kingdom', *Bioethics*, 11 (1997), pp. 277–90.

Singer, Peter, *Practical Ethics*, 2nd ed., (Cambridge: Cambridge University, 1993).

_____, *Animal Liberation*, (London: Jonathon Cape, 1975).

Singer et al. (eds), *Embryo Experimentation*, (Melbourne: Cambridge University, 1990).

Singer, Peter and Dawson, Karen, 'IVF Technology and the Argument from Potential', in Singer et al. (eds), *Embryo Experimentation*, (Melbourne: Cambridge University, 1990).

Singer, Peter and Wells, Deane, *The Reproduction Revolution: New Ways of Making Babies*, (Oxford: Oxford University, 1984). Revised North American edition published as *Making Babies: The New Science and Ethics of Conception*, (New York: Scribners, 1985).

Sinnott–Armstrong, Walter, 'You Can't Lose What You Ain't Never Had: A Reply to Marquis on Abortion', *Philosophical Studies*, 96 (1997), pp. 59–72.

Smart, Carol, *Feminism and the Power of Law*, (London: Routledge, 1989), p. 153.

Smart, C. and Sevenhuijsen, S., (eds), *Child Custody and the Politics of Gender*, (London: Routledge, 1989).

Squier, Susan Merrill, *Babies in Bottles: Twentieth-Century Visions of Reproductive Technology*, (New Brunswick: Rutgers, 1994).

Steinbock, Bonnie, *Life Before Birth: The Moral and Legal Status of Embryos and Foetuses*, (New York: Oxford University, 1992).

Stith, Richard, 'A Secular Case Against Abortion', in Garry Brodsky, John Troyer and David Vance (eds), *Contemporary Readings in Social and Political Ethics*, (Buffalo: Prometheus, 1984).

Stone, Jim, 'Why Potentiality Matters', *Canadian Journal of Philosophy*, 17 (1987), pp. 815–30.

Sumner, L. W., 'A Third Way', in Susan Dwyer and Joel Feinberg (eds), *The Problem of Abortion*, 3rd ed., (Belmont CA: Wadsworth, 1997).

Therkelsen, Aage J. et al., 'Ethics and Medical Genetics in Denmark', in Dorothy C. Wertz and John C. Fletcher (eds), *Ethics and Human Genetics*, (1989), pp. 141–55.

Thomson, Judith Jarvis, 'A Defence of Abortion', *Philosophy and Public Affairs*, 1 (1971), pp. 47–66.

Tooley, Michael, 'Abortion and Infanticide', *Philosophy and Public Affairs*, 2 (1972), pp. 37–65.

Uniacke, Suzanne, '*In Vitro* Fertilisation and the Right to Reproduce', *Bioethics*, 1 (1987), pp. 241–54.

US Immigration and Naturalization Service, 'INS Decision in the Elian Gonzalez Case', 5 January 2000.

Victorian Infertility Treatment Act, 1995 Act No. 63/1995, as amended 1/1/98.

Walters, William A., 'The Artificial Induction of Abdominal Pregnancy' in *Bailliere's Clinical Obstetrics and Gynaecology: International Practice and Research – Human Reproduction: Current and Future Ethical Issues*, 5 (1991), pp. 731–41.

Warnock, Mary, *A Question of Life: The Warnock Report on Human Fertilisation and Embryology*, (Oxford: Basil Blackwell, 1985).

Warren, Mary Anne, *Moral Status: Obligations to Persons and Other Living Things*, (Oxford: Oxford University, 1997).

_____, 'The Moral Significance of Birth', *Hypatia*, 4 (1989), pp. 46–65.

_____, 'On the Moral and Legal Status of Abortion', in R. Wasserstrom (ed.), *Today's Moral Problems*, (New York: MacMillan, 1975).

Wells, Deane, 'Ectogenesis, Justice and Utility: A Reply to James', *Bioethics*, 1 (1987), pp. 372–79.

Wendler, Dave, 'Understanding the "Conservative" View on Abortion', *Bioethics*, 13 (1999), pp. 32–56.

Wreen, Michael J., 'The Power of Potentiality', *Theoria*, 52 (1986), pp. 16–40.

Yasuda, Y. et al., 'Foetus-in-Foetu; Report of a Case', *Teratology*, 31 (1985), pp. 337–41.

Yeung, Anthony Kwok-Wing, 'Mere Potential Persons and Developing Potential Persons' presented at the International Conference on Applied Ethics, Hong Kong, December 1999.

Yu, V.Y.H., 'Prematurity and Low Birth Weight'. in Robinson and Roberton (eds), *Practical Paediatrics*, 4th ed., (Edinburgh: Churchill Livingstone, 1998).

_____, 'Improving the Outcome of Preterm and Low Birthweight Infants', unpublished manuscript, (1995).

Zapol, Warren et al., 'Extracorporeal Membrane Oxygenation in Severe Acute Respiratory Failure: A Randomised Prospective Study', *Journal of the American Medical Association*, 242 (1979), p. 2193.

_____, 'Artificial Placenta: Two Days of Extrauterine Support of the Isolated Premature Lamb Foetus', *Science*, 166 (1969), pp. 617–8.

Index